Lawrence Robbins



# Advanced Headache Therapy

## Outpatient Strategies

Springer

Lawrence Robbins
Robbins Headache Clinic
Riverwoods
Illinois
USA

ISBN 978-3-319-13898-5 ISBN 978-3-319-13899-2 (eBook)
DOI 10.1007/978-3-319-13899-2

Library of Congress Control Number: 2015930452

Springer Cham Heidelberg New York Dordrecht London


Printed on acid-free paper

Springer is part of Springer Science+Business Media (www.springer.com)

# Preface

This book fills a need for a practical guide to advanced headache management. Headache patients are complicated, often with medical and/or psychiatric comorbidities. I provide an in-depth analysis of options for refractory "difficult-to-treat" patients. Management of the routine in easier headache patient is also included. Most of this book was written in late 2014; there are a few older articles that did not require an update.

I wrote this for physicians and patients who have an interest in headache. The style is simple, so that patients find the material to be understandable. Physicians specializing in headache will find this material practical and cutting-edge. Patients with refractory, difficult headaches will learn about strategies for when "nothing has worked."

Chapter 1 is a complete guide to migraine management. Non-medicine strategies are outlined, along with an extensive discussion of the medications. The chapter is infused with my philosophies on treating headache such as "comorbidities drive where we go with medications." An extensive clinical pearls section gives many practical tips not found elsewhere.

I then focus on refractory topics, including a complete guide to outpatient management of refractory headache. Opioids, stimulants, the use of daily triptans, SPG and occipital blocks, Botox, and MAOI's are among the topics analyzed. Chapter 3 provides a blueprint for treating children and adolescents. There is a discourse on approaches to the refractory adolescent who is not attending school. A dialogue on factitious disorder by proxy is included, with management suggestions. Cluster headache management of both routine and refractory patients is thoroughly addressed. A typical cluster case study is explored. Chapter 5 focuses on psychiatric comorbidities. Anxiety and attention deficit hyperactivity disorder (ADHD) in the headache patient are examined. There is an extensive discourse on the bipolar spectrum and personality disorders, and how they affect headache management. Three interactive case studies are presented. They follow one young patient with multiple comorbidities over a 10-year span. The miscellaneous section contains sections on new daily persistent headache (NDPH) as well as the immune system and headache. Handouts on exercise and supplements for headache patients are also included.

Legal note: This book is not meant to be prescriptive. These are the opinions of this author and are not meant to represent "standard" therapy. Risk/benefit and informed consent must be addressed between the patient and physician. All medications have possible adverse events and the patient should understand and accept those possible side effects.

Northbrook, Ill. Lawrence Robbins
Chicagoheadacheclinic.com; lrobb98@aol.com

# Contents

# About the Author

**Lawrence Robbins MD** is a neurologist and headache specialist in Northbrook, Ill. He has written three books on headache previously, two out in 2nd editions. The books are: Management of Headache and Headache Medications, Headache Help, and an e-book, Headache 2013.

Dr. Robbins has written more than 250 articles and abstracts, mostly on headache subjects. He has a special interest in refractory "difficult-to-treat" headaches. Dr. Robbins started the section of the American Headache Society "Refractory Headache" in 2001, and has published extensively on refractory headache.

In 2008 Dr. Robbins was awarded the "Janet Travell" clinical award by the American Academy of Pain Management. Dr. Robbins was on staff at the University of Illinois neurology department, and also was an assistant professor of neurology at Rush Medical College. www.chicagoheadacheclinic.com. E-mail: lrobb98@aol.com.

# Chapter 1
# Migraine and Headache: General

## Migraine Treatment: 2015–2016

Migraine is a very common and disabling illness. Choosing a therapeutic agent that is best for each individual patient requires consideration of the patient's history, lifestyle, comorbid conditions, and individual preferences.

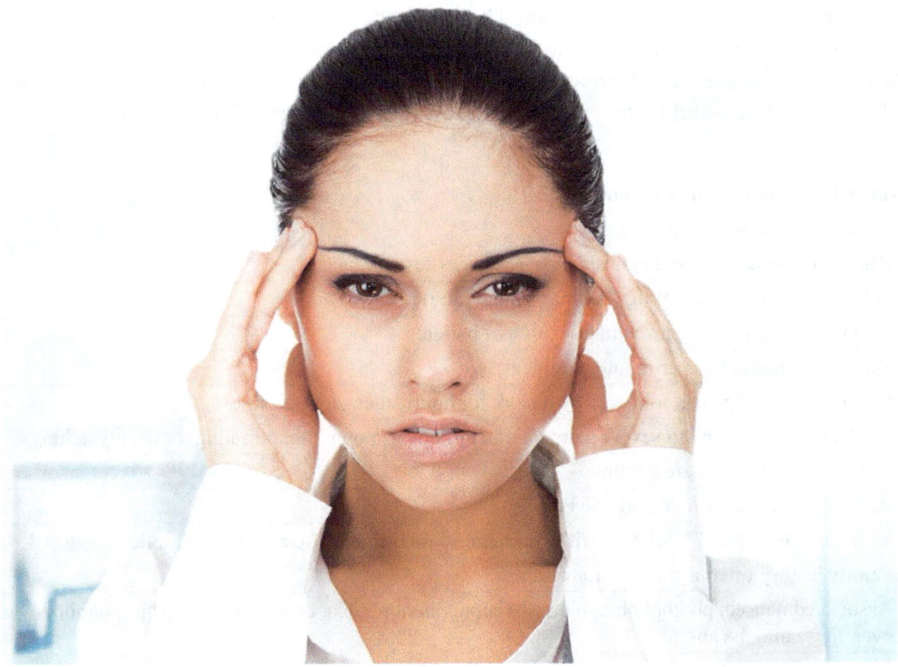



L. Robbins, *Advanced Headache Therapy*, DOI 10.1007/978-3-319-13899-2_1

Migraine headaches are a common cause of disability in the USA, affecting approximately 25 to 28 million American adults, or 18% of women and 7% of men [6]. To help define migraines better, the term classical migraine has been replaced with migraine with aura, and nonclassical migraine now is referred to as migraine without aura. Chronic migraine, which affects 3.2 million Americans (2%), is defined as having migraine symptoms for at least 15 days per month, lasting at least 4 h, and for longer than 3 months in duration. This is in contrast to episodic migraine, which causes symptoms on fewer than 15 days per month [4]. Current treatment for chronic migraine is divided into acute abortive agents (analgesics, triptans, ergots, etc.) and medications to prevent migraine onset.

This chapter highlights the current definition of migraines as well as treatment options.

## *Migraine Characteristics*

A recurring headache that is of moderate or severe intensity and is triggered by migraine-precipitating factors usually is considered to be migraine. Precipitating factors can include stress, certain foods, weather changes, smoke, hunger, fatigue, hormones, and so on. Migraine without aura is a chronic idiopathic headache disorder with attacks lasting 4–72 h. Status migrainosus applies to migraine headaches that exceed 72 h. Migraine features often include a unilateral location and a throbbing or pulsating nature to the pain. There may be associated nausea, photophobia, phonophobia, or dizziness (Table 1.1). Further characteristics include a positive relationship with menses, decreased frequency during pregnancy, increased pain with physical activity, and history of migraine in first-degree relatives. Between 70 and

**Table 1.1** Characteristics of a migraine

| |
|---|
| Attacks last from 4–72 h |
| Patient history gives the diagnosis (not laboratory tests) |
| Often occur in early morning (but may be anytime) |
| Unilateral location in approximately 50% of patients |
| One to five migraines per month is typical |
| Gradual onset of pain is followed by a peak for hours, then slow decline |
| Moderate or moderate to severe pain; pain is throbbing, pounding, pulsating, or deeply aching |
| Sharp "ice-pick" jabs are common |
| Peak ages are between 20 and 35 years |
| 18% of women and 7% of men will experience a migraine in their lifetime; female ratio is 3:1 |
| Family history often is positive for migraine |
| Associated nausea, photophobia, blurred vision, phonophobia, or dizziness are common; however, these may be absent |
| In women, there often is a positive relationship with menses |
| Cold hands and feet and motion sickness are common |

75 % of migraine patients report that they have a first-degree relative with a history of migraines [3].

Patients who suffer from migraines often have colder hands and feet compared with controls, and the prevalence of motion sickness is much higher in migraine patients. Although most patients will not have all of these characteristics, there are certain diagnostic criteria that have been established by the International Headache Society for the definitive diagnosis of migraine [4]. Distinguishing a milder migraine without aura from a moderate or severe tension headache may be difficult, and it is not surprising when "pure" migraine medications are effective for severe tension-type headaches.

## Taking a History

The patient's history is used to make the diagnosis of migraine. Physical examination and magnetic resonance imaging (MRI) or computed tomography (CT) scans are helpful only in ruling out organic pathology. Recent-onset headaches need to be investigated with an MRI scan to rule out other organic disorders, particularly brain tumors. In addition to physical exam and imaging, a check of intraocular pressure (IOP) may be warranted. With new-onset headaches, an eye exam is always warranted.

Although the pain is unilateral in 50 % of migraine patients, the entire head often becomes involved. The pain may be in the facial or the cervical areas, and often will shift sides from one occurrence to another. Most patients, however, suffer the severe pain on one favored side from attack to attack.

The typical migraine patient suffers 1–5 attacks in a month, but many patients average less than 1 (episodic) or more than 10 per month (chronic). The attack frequency varies with the seasons, and many patients can identify a time of year when their headaches increase significantly. Patients with chronic migraine may have 15 days a month of headache, and many even have 30 days per month, with pain described as 24/7.

The pain of the migraine often follows a bell-shaped curve, with a gradual ascent, a peak for a number of hours, and then a slow decline (Table 1.2). Occasionally, the pain may be at its peak within minutes of onset. Many patients with migraine suffer some degree of nausea during the attack, and many patients experience vomiting as well. The nausea is often mild, and some patients are not bothered by it. Many patients state that the headache is lessened after they vomit. Diarrhea may occur and usually is mild to moderate. The presence of diarrhea renders the use of rectal suppositories impossible. Light-headedness often accompanies the migraine, and syncope may occur. Most patients become very sensitive to bright lights (photophobia), sounds (phonophobia), and/or odors. Between migraine attacks, many patients retain the photophobia, and it is common for migraine patients to wear sunglasses most of the time. Sensitivity to bright lights is a distinctive migraine characteristic.

**Table 1.2** Somatic symptoms

| Accompanying migraine[a] |
| --- |
| Sensitivity to light (photophobia) |
| Blurred vision |
| Nausea |
| Sensitivity to noise (phonophobia) |
| Scalp tenderness |
| Dizziness or light-headedness |
| Lethargy |
| Vomiting |
| Sensitivity to odors |
| Retention of fluid, with weight gain |
| Photopsia (light flashes/flickers) |
| Vertigo |
| Anxiety |
| Paresthesias (numbness/tingling) |
| Diarrhea |
| Fortification spectra |
| Nasal stuffiness |
| Mild aphasia (slurred speech) |
| Syncope or near syncope |
| Severe confusion |
| Seizures |
| Fever |
| Hemiparesis or hemiplegia |
| Ataxia or dysarthria (brainstem dysfunction) |

[a]Listed in order of frequency

Pallor of the face is common during a migraine; flushing may occur as well but is seen less often. Patients complain of feeling excessively hot or cold during an attack, and the skin temperature may increase or decrease on the side with pain. Patients with migraines often experience tenderness of the scalp that may linger for hours or days after the migraine pain has ceased. This tenderness actually may occur during the prodrome of the migraine. Both vascular and muscular factors contribute to the scalp tenderness. Autonomic disturbances, such as pupillary miosis or dilation, runny nose, eye tearing, and nasal stuffiness, are relatively common. These also are symptoms of cluster headache, including the sharp pain about one eye or temple.

Alterations of mood are seen in many patients before, during, and after migraine attacks. Patients are usually anxious, tired, or depressed. They often feel "washed out" after an attack, but a calm or an euphoric state occasionally is seen as a postdrome to the migraine. Rarely, euphoria or exhilaration may precede a migraine.

Weight gain due to fluid retention may occur prior to the onset of the migraine. The weight gain is usually less than 6 lb, and is transient.

At some point during the migraine, patients often experience polyuria.

## *Visual Disturbances*

Approximately 25% of patients experience visual or other neurologic symptoms preceding or during the migraine; these auras may be as disturbing to the patient as the migraine pain itself. The visual symptoms usually last 15–20 min, and most often will be followed by the migraine headache. Most migraine sufferers experience the same aura with each migraine, but, occasionally, one person may have several types of auras. "The light of a flashbulb going off" is the description many patients give to describe their aura. The visual hallucinations seen most often consist of spots, stars, lines (often wavy), color splashes, and waves resembling heat waves. The images may seem to shimmer, sparkle, or flicker. These visual occurrences are referred to as photopsia. Fortification spectra are seen much less often than photopsia. They usually begin with a decrease in vision and visual hallucinations that are unformed. Within minutes, a paracentral scotoma becomes evident and assumes a crescent shape, usually with zigzags. There often is associated shimmering, sparkling, or flickering at the edges of the scotoma. Patients may experience a "graying out" of their vision, or a "white out" may occur. Some patients suffer complete visual loss, usually for some minutes. Photopsia may be experienced at the same time as the gray out, white out, or visual loss.

## *Miscellaneous Neurologic Symptoms*

Numbness or tingling (paresthesias) commonly are experienced by patients as part of a migraine. These are experienced most often in one hand and forearm, but may be felt in the face, periorally, or in both arms and legs. Like the visual disturbances, they often last only minutes preceding the pain, but the numbness may continue for hours, and at times the paresthesias are severe. The sensory disturbances usually increase slowly over 15–25 min, differentiating them from those with a more rapid pace that are seen in epilepsy.

Paralysis of the limbs may occur, but this is rare. This occasionally is seen as a familial autosomal dominant trait, which is termed familial hemiplegic migraine. With the weakness, aphasia or slurred speech may also occur, and sensory disturbances are seen ipsilateral to the weakness.

Vertigo occasionally is experienced during migraine, and may be disabling.

"Migraine-associated vertigo" has become a common diagnosis. Ataxia may occur, but it is not common. Rarely, multiple symptoms of brain stem dysfunction occur, with the term migraine with brainstem aura (previously called basilar migraine) being applied to this type of syndrome. The attack usually begins with visual disturbances (most often photopsia), followed by ataxia, vertigo, paresthesias, and other brain stem symptoms. These severe neurologic symptoms usually abate after 15–30 min and are followed by a headache. This type of migraine often stops over months or years, and the patient is simply left with migraine headaches without neurologic dysfunction.

## *Workup for Migraine*

As noted, when patients present with a long history of typical migraine attacks, and the headaches are essentially unchanged, scans of the head may not be necessary. Whether to do any testing at all depends on the physician's clinical suspicion of organic pathology. Sound clinical judgment, based on patient history and a physical exam, is crucial in deciding which exams a given patient needs.

In addition to the MRI and CT scan, tests that are generally useful for diagnosis of headache include lumbar puncture, IOP testing, CT scan of the sinuses, and blood tests. A magnetic resonance angiogram (MRA) allows the detection of most intracranial aneurysms.

The problems that need to be excluded in a patient with new-onset migraine include sinus disease, meningitis, glaucoma, brain tumor, arteritis, subarachnoid hemorrhage, idiopathic intracranial hypertension, hydrocephalus, pheochromocytoma, stroke or transient ischemic attack, internal carotid artery dissection, and systemic illness.

**Situations that raise concern about organic pathology include:**

- Progressive headaches over days or weeks, increasing in intensity
- New-onset headaches, particularly in patients who "never" get headaches, or new-onset exertional headaches
- Neurologic symptoms or signs, stiff neck, papilledema, and changes in level of consciousness
- A fever that is not explained
- Radical increase or change in a preexisting headache pattern

## *Headache Triggers*

With migraine and chronic daily headache sufferers, avoidance of triggers should be emphasized. The most common triggers are stress (both during and after stress), weather changes, perimenstruation, missing meals, bright lights or sunlight, under- and oversleeping, food sensitivity, perfume, cigarette smoke, exercise, and sexual activity. Some foods can be headache triggers, but foods tend to be overemphasized. In general, headache patients do better with regular schedules, eating three or more meals per day, and going to bed and awaking at the same time every day. Many patients state that "I can tell the weather with my head." Barometric changes and storms are typical weather culprits, but some patients do poorly on bright "sunglare" days.

Regarding stress as a trigger, it is not so much extreme stress but rather daily hassles that increase headaches. When patients are faced with overwhelming daily stress, particularly when they are not sleeping well at night, headaches can be much worse the next day.

Psychotherapy is extremely useful for many headache patients with regard to stress management, coping, life issues, family-of-origin issues, and so on. Although psychotherapy may be recommended, it is crucial to legitimize the headaches as a physical condition; headaches are not a "psychological" problem but rather a physical one that stress may exacerbate. If a person inherits the brain chemistry for headache, these triggers come into play; without the inherited genetics, most people may have stress/weather changes/hormonal changes but not experience a headache.

Managing stress with exercise, yoga, and Pilates, often will reduce the frequency of headaches. The ideal would be for the patient to take a class weekly, then do the stretches and breathing for 10 min/day. Relaxation techniques such as biofeedback, deep breathing, and imaging also can be helpful for daily headache patients, particularly when stress is a factor.

Many migraine patients have accompanying neck pain. Physical therapy may help, and acupuncture or chiropractic treatments occasionally help as well. Certain physical therapists "specialize" in head and neck pain. Massage may be effective, but the relief often is short-lived. Temporomandibular disorder (TMD), with clenching and/or bruxing, may exacerbate migraine. For patients with TMD, physical therapy, a bite splint, and/or onobotulinum toxin A (Botox) injections may help. It often "takes a village" to help a person with pain, and we recruit other "villagers," such as physical therapists and psychotherapists.

## Caffeine Use

Although caffeine can help headaches, overuse may increase headaches. Patients must limit total caffeine intake from all sources (e.g., coffee, caffeine pills, or combination analgesics). The maximum amount of caffeine taken each day varies from person to person, depending on sleep patterns, presence of anxiety, and sensitivity to possible rebound headaches. In general, caffeine should be limited to no more than 150 or 200 mg/day (Table 1.3).

## Foods to Avoid

As noted, multiple food sensitivities are not common. Patients tend to focus on food, because it is a tangible trigger that one can control (as opposed to weather, for example). However, most people are sensitive to only two or three types of food in the diet. If a particular food is going to cause a headache, it usually will occur within 3 h of eating that food. Table 1.4 provides a list of foods to avoid.

**Table 1.3** Common caffeine sources and content[a]

| |
|---|
| Brewed coffee: 75–150 mg/8 oz (cup). Drip is the strongest form, percolated is weaker. Coffee from specialty brewers, such as Starbucks, may be up to 50 % stronger than home brewed. A small latte has 70–90 mg of caffeine |
| Instant coffee: 40–150 mg/8 oz, usually closer to 40 mg |
| Decaf coffee: about 5 mg/8 oz, but may be higher |
| Tea: 30–50 mg/8 oz |
| Soft drinks: approximately 40 mg/8 oz; energy drinks may have more than 200 mg/8 oz |
| Chocolate: 1–15 mg/oz |
| Cocoa: 20–50 mg/8 oz |
| Caffeine tablets: (NoDoz, Vivarin, Tirend) contain 100 mg of caffeine |
| Caffeine also is present in many analgesic medications, such as Excedrin Migraine (65 mg), Anacin (32 mg), and Vanquish (33 mg) |

[a]Limit caffeine to 150 mg/day, or at most 200 mg/day

**Table 1.4** Foods to avoid

| |
|---|
| Monosodium glutamate (MSG)—also labeled as autolyzed yeast extract, hydrolyzed vegetable protein, or natural flavoring. Possible sources of MSG include broths or soup stocks; seasonings; whey protein; soy extract; malt extract; caseinate; barley extract; textured soy protein; chicken, pork, or beef flavoring; meat tenderizer; smoke flavor; spices, carrageenan; seasoned salt; TV dinners; instant gravies; and some potato chips and dry-roasted nuts |
| Alcohol. All alcohol can trigger a headache; beer and red wine are the worst offenders. White wine is not as likely to trigger a headache |
| Cheese. Ripened, aged cheeses (Colby, Cheddar, Roquefort, Brie, Gruyere, bleu, Boursault, mozzarella, Parmesan, Romano) and processed cheese are the worst. Less likely to trigger a headache: cottage cheese, cream cheese, and American cheese |
| Chocolate |
| Citrus fruits |
| Meat that has been cured or processed, such as bacon, bologna, ham, hot dogs, pepperoni, salami, sausage; canned, aged, or marinated meats |
| Nuts, peanut butter |
| Yogurt, sour cream |
| Large amounts of aspartame (NutraSweet) |

## *Medications: Abortives*

The most common first-line treatment for migraines includes triptans. More than 200 million patients worldwide have used triptans. The most effective way to use triptans is to take them early in the headache—the earlier a patient takes these agents, the better the effect. Sumatriptan is an extremely effective migraine-abortive medication with minimal side effects. It is effective for approximately 70 % of patients and has become the gold standard in abortive headache treatment. The usual dose is one tablet every 3 h, as needed; maximum dose, two tablets per day.

However, clinicians do need to limit triptan use (ideally, 3 days per week) to avoid rebound headaches or medication overuse headaches (MOH).

Triptans are helpful for moderate as well as more severe migraines. Certain patients may tolerate one triptan better than others, and it is worthwhile for patients to try several. Triptans are an excellent choice for migraine patients who are not at risk for coronary artery disease (CAD). Patients in their 50s or 60s can use these drugs, but they should be prescribed cautiously, and only in those patients who have been screened for CAD. Over the 23 years that triptans have been available, serious side effects have been few; they appear to be much safer than was previously thought in 1993.

As noted, if patients do not do well with one triptan (lack of efficacy or side effects), it is usually worthwhile for them to try at least one or two other triptans. While they are all very similar, the minor chemical differences between them mean that some patients do well with one, and not another.

The usual triptan side effects may include pressure (or tightness) in the chest/neck (or other muscle areas), tingling, and fatigue. These are usually transient, lasting 10–30 min. If a patient experiences moderate to severe chest/throat/neck pressure (or pain), we usually discontinue the triptan or substitute a milder one (naratriptan/frovatriptan). The chest symptoms are rarely cardiac in nature, which is the primary concern with chest symptoms.

There are a number of triptan choices. Sumatriptan, zolmitriptan, rizatriptan, and naratriptan are available in generic formulations. Eletripton (Relpax) is a very effective triptan and almotriptan (Axert) is useful for many patients (Fig. 1.1).

Treximet is a combination of sumatriptan and naproxen. Frovatriptan (Frova) is a "slow onset," milder triptan, which has a longer half-life. Zolmitriptan (Zomig) nasal spray is not generic, but it is very effective, with a quick onset of action. The sumatriptan injections (available in various forms) remain the most effective migraine abortives.

For patients who cannot tolerate triptans, there are a number of other effective nontriptan first-line approaches, including diclofenac potassium powder (Cambia), Excedrin Migraine, naproxen, ketorolac, ibuprofen, and Prodrin (similar to Midrin, but without the sedative). We often combine two first-line approaches—for example, a triptan and a nonsteroidal anti-inflammatory drug (NSAID).

In general, drugs containing ergotamine (also called ergots) are effective second-line therapy for migraines. They were the first antimigraine drugs available, but they have many side effects, and, at most, should be used only 2 days per week. Dihydroergotamine (DHE) is the safest ergot derivative. Intravenous DHE primarily is a "venoconstrictor" with few arterial effects. This renders it very unlikely to cause cardiac problems. Indeed, since its introduction in 1945, DHE has been remarkably safe. Intravenous DHE can be administered in the office or emergency room. Nasal (Migranal Nasal Spray) and inhaled forms of DHE (soon to be released) have been found to be safe and effective as well.

Barbiturates and opioids have been studied and are effective, but because of the risk for addiction, they should be used sparingly. For severe prolonged migraines, corticosteroids (oral, intravenous (IV), or intramuscular) often are effective. It is important to use low doses of steroids.

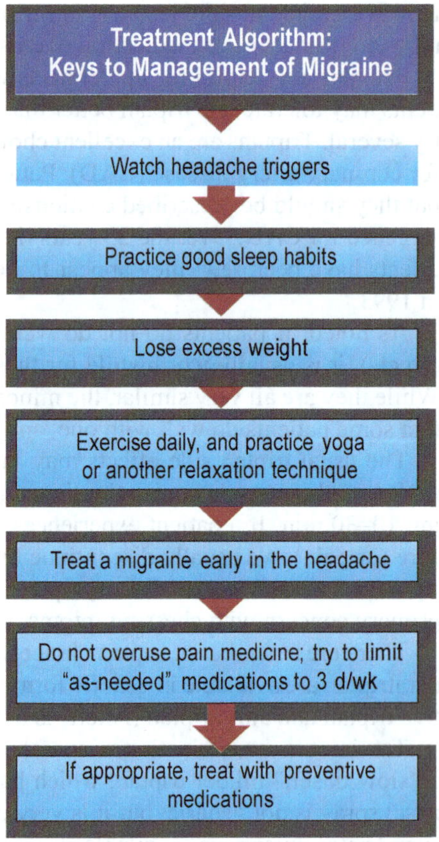


**Fig. 1.1** Management tips for patients

Many patients use 3–6 abortives: a triptan, NSAID, Excedrin, an antinausea medication, and a painkiller (opioid/butalbital). Patients will use each medication in different situations, for different types and degrees of headache. Tables 1.5, 1.6, and 1.7 review all the first- and second-line migraine-abortive medications.

## *Miscellaneous Approaches*

Muscle relaxants (carisoprodol, diazepam) or tranquilizers (clonazepam, alprazolam) occasionally are useful, primarily to aid in sleeping. Intravenous valproate sodium (Depacon) is safe and can be effective. The atypical antipsychotics, such as olanzapine (Zyprexa) or quetiapine (Seroquel), occasionally may be useful on an as-needed basis. In the emergency room, IV administration of antiemetic agents such as prochlorperazine (Compazine, others) or metoclopramide (Reglan) may be useful (Table 1.8). Certain preventive medications, such as valproic acid, or divalproex sodium (Depakote), topiramate (Topamax), and amitriptyline—in low doses every 4–6 h—may be useful on an as-needed basis. The antihistamine diphenhydr-

**Table 1.5** First-line abortive medications: Triptans[a]

| Drug name (brand) | Formulations | Usual dosage | Comments |
|---|---|---|---|
| Almotriptan (Axert) | Oral tablet | 12.5 mg every 3–4 h; limit to 25 mg/day | Similar to other triptans, almotriptan combines good efficacy with excellent tolerability. In 2009, almotriptan gained an official FDA indication for use in adolescents with migraine |
| Eletriptan (Relpax) | Oral tablet | 40 mg every 4 h; limit to 80 mg/day | Effective and well tolerated; minimal side effects include nausea, pressure in the throat, dizziness, and tiredness or weakness |
| Frovatriptan (Frova) | Oral tablet | 2.5 mg every 4 h; limit to 5 mg/day | Useful for slower-onset moderate or moderate to severe migraines; effective for preventing menstrual migraines<br>Long (26 h) half-life advantageous for patients with prolonged migraines. Mean maximal blood concentrations are seen approximately 2–4 h after a dose |
| Naratriptan (Amerge, generic) | Oral tablet | 1 tablet every 3–4 h; maximum 2 doses per day | Milder, longer-acting triptan. A generic form is available |
| Rizatriptan (Maxalt, generic) | Oral tablet and rapidly disintegrating tablet | 10 mg every 4 h; maximum 3 doses per day | Similar to sumatriptan (see below). Maxalt MLT (rapidly disintegrating tablets) is placed on the tongue; tablets have a pleasant taste and may be taken without water<br>Approved for use in children and adolescents<br>Side effects are similar to those of sumatriptan. A generic form is available |
| Sumatriptan (Imitrex, generic) | Oral tablet and nasal spray, a skin patch will be available Zecuity (for age 18 and up) is a unique sumatriptan skin patch, 6.5mg (low dose) over 4 hours; bypassing the GI tract, Zecuity has a good niche | Oral: 50 and 100 mg tablet every 2–3 h; maximum 200 mg/day<br>Nasal spray: maximum daily dose, 40 mg | More than 100 million people have used sumatriptan over the past 20 years. The generic form of sumatriptan is the least expensive triptan available |

**Table 1.5** (continued)

| Drug name (brand) | Formulations | Usual dosage | Comments |
|---|---|---|---|
| Sumatriptan (Imitrex STAT-dose, Sumavel DosePro, Alsuma, or generic prefilled syringes) | Subcutaneous injection | Injection: 4 and 6 mg every 3–4 h as needed; maximum dosing: twice daily\| | Although the usual dose had been 6 mg, the 4 mg STAT dose often is effective. A generic STAT form is available. Sumavel is a good "needle-free" option<br>Alsuma is a new "EpiPen" device containing 6 mg/0.5 mL of sumatriptan. A generic form is available<br>There are also generic, easy-to-use prefilled syringes of 6 mg sumatriptan |
| Sumatriptan plus naproxen (Treximet) | Oral tablet | 85 mg sumatriptan and 500 mg naproxen sodium. Dosage: 1 tablet every 3–4 h; maximum daily dose: 2 tablets | Treximet is an excellent combination drug that helps prevent recurrence of headache. The addition of naproxen may cause stomach pain or nausea |
| Zolmitriptan (Zomig, generic tablets; Zomig 5 mg nasal spray) | Dissolvable tablet and nasal spray | Oral: 2.5 or 5 mg; usual dose 5 mg every 3–4 h as needed; maximum 10 mg/day<br>Nasal spray: 2.5 or 5 mg | Zolmitriptan ZMT, 5 mg, is a pleasant-tasting, dissolvable tablet. Like Maxalt MLT, it provides an alternative to the oral tablets. A generic ZMT form is available<br>The nasal spray is very effective, works quickly |

*FDA* Food and Drug Administration, *NSAID* nonsteroidal anti-inflammatory drug
[a] All FDA-approved for migraine. The addition of an NSAID to a triptan may enhance efficacy and prevent recurrence

**Table 1.6** First-line abortives for migraine: nontriptans

| Drug name (brand) | FDA-approved for migraines | Formulations | Dosage | Comments |
|---|---|---|---|---|
| Acetaminophen-containing products | | | | |
| Excedrin migraine | Yes | Oral tablet | Usual dose: 1–2 tablets every 3 h; maximum of 4 tablets per day<br>Tablets contain 250 mg aspirin, 65 mg caffeine, and 250 mg acetaminophen | Useful OTC for patients with mild or moderate migraines. Anxiety from the caffeine and nausea from the aspirin is common<br>Rebound headache may occur with overuse; 4 tablets per day (but not on a daily basis) should be maximum. Patients need to be educated about not exceeding acetaminophen's upper daily limits |

**Table 1.6** (continued)

| Drug name (brand) | FDA-approved for migraines | Formulations | Dosage | Comments |
|---|---|---|---|---|
| Prodrin | Yes | Oral tablet | Usual dose: 1 tablet every 2–3 h; limit to 2–3 doses per day<br>Tablets contain 20 mg caffeine, 65 mg isometheptene, and 325 mg acetaminophen | Nonsedating and nonaddictive. Caffeine may cause nervousness or a faster heartbeat; limit dosing to 2–3 times per day<br>Patients with insomnia should not use Prodrin after 3 p.m. Patients with hypertension should use with caution, and only if blood pressure is controlled<br>If not available, generic Midrin, which has a sedative and no caffeine, usually is used, along with additional caffeine<br>Patients need to be educated about not exceeding acetaminophen's upper daily limits |
| *NSAIDs* | | | | |
| Diclofenac potassium powder (Cambia) | Yes | Packets dissolved in water. Available in boxes of 3 or 9 packets | 50-mg packet every 2–4 h, maximum dose 150 mg/day | Excellent new migraine abortive. Useful in younger patients and in older individuals who can tolerate NSAIDs. Typical side effects of NSAIDs, primarily GI, may occur<br>May be combined with triptans; caffeine may be added to increase efficacy |
| Ibuprofen (Advil, Motrin, generic) | No | Liquid and oral tablet/capsule | 400–800 mg every 3 h; maximum dose 2400 mg/day | Available OTC and approved for children; occasionally useful in treating menstrual migraine. GI side effects are common<br>May be used with triptans; caffeine increases efficacy |
| Naproxen (Anaprox, Aleve, generic) | No | Oral tablet and capsule | 220 mg; usual dose, 500 mg, repeated in 1 h and again 3–4 h; maximum dose 1000 mg/day | Useful in younger patients; occasionally helpful for menstrual migraine. Nonsedating, but patients frequently report GI upset. First/usual dose is taken with food or a Tums; may be repeated in 1 h if no severe nausea is present, and again in 3–4 h<br>May be used with triptans; caffeine increases efficacy |

*GI* gastrointestinal, *NSAID* nonsteroidal anti-inflammatory drug, *OTC* over the counter

**Table 1.7** Second-line abortive medications for migraine

| Drug name (brand) | Formulations | Usual dosage | Comments |
|---|---|---|---|
| NSAIDs | | | |
| Ketorolac (Toradol, generic; Sprix nasal spray) | Oral, IM, nasal spray | Injection: 60 mg/2 mL; repeat in 4 h if needed. Maximum dose, 2 injections per day<br>Oral: 2 tablets per day, at most | Ketorolac intramuscular (IM) injections, which can be administered at home, are much more effective than tablets. Nausea or GI pain may occur. Ketorolac is nonaddicting and does not usually cause sedation. Limit to 3 injections per week due to possible nephrotoxicity. IV ketorolac is very effective<br>There is a new nasal spray form of ketorolac (Sprix), which may produce a burning feeling in the throat. Sprix is more effective than tablets but not as effective as IM |
| *DHE* | | | |
| Dihydroergotamine (Migranal nasal spray, generic DHE) | IV, IM, nasal Spray and an inhaled version will be available | 1 mg IM or IV; may be titrated up or down<br>If it is the first time a patient has used DHE, start with 0.33 or 0.50 mL only | Effective as an IV or IM injection, and may be effective as a nasal spray. Migranal is the brand name of DHE nasal spray; inhaled form of DHE is awaiting FDA approval<br>All forms of DHE are safe and well tolerated. Nausea, leg cramps, and burning at the injection side are common. IV DHE is very effective in the office or emergency room. Less likely to cause MOH than many other abortives |
| *Butalbital* | | | |
| Butalbital (Phrenilin) Butalbital, aspirin and caffeine (Fiorinal)<br>Butalbital, acetaminophen, and caffeine (Fioricet, Esgic)<br>Butalbital, acetaminophen, caffeine, and 30 mg codeine (Fiorinal #3) | Oral tablets and capsules | 1–2 tablets or capsules every 3 h; maximum dose, 4 tablets per day. Limit to 30 or 40 pills per month | Barbiturate medications are addicting but very effective for many patients. Generics of these compounds may not work as well<br>Fiorinal #3 is more effective than plain Fiorinal or Fioricet<br>Phrenilin contains no aspirin or caffeine and is very useful at night and in those with GI upset. Brief fatique and spacey or euphoric feelings are common side effects<br>Butalbital must be used sparingly in younger people. MOH is always a concern with butalbital and opioids |

**Table 1.7** (continued)

| Drug name (brand) | Formulations | Usual dosage | Comments |
|---|---|---|---|
| *Opioids* | | | |
| Hydrocodone and acetaminophen (Vicodin, Norco, generic)<br>Hydrocodone and ibuprofen (Vicoprofen)<br>Oxycodone (generic) Meperidine (generic) Tramadol (Ultram) | Oral, IM | See individual PIs. These must be limited per day, and per month | By mouth or IM, opioids often are the best of the "last resort" approaches. When given IM, they usually are combined with an antiemetic<br>Although addiction is a potential problem, it is crucial to understand the difference between dependency and addiction<br>Tramadol is milder, with relatively few side effects<br>Hydrocodone is now Schedule II, limiting access<br>Vicoprofen is more effective than the other hydrocodone preparations because of the addition of ibuprofen and, generally, is well tolerated |
| *Corticosteroids* | | | |
| Cortisone (generic)<br>Dexamethasone (Decadron)<br>Prednisone (generic) | Oral, IV, and IM | Dexamethasone: 4 mg (½ to 1 tablet) every 8–12 h as needed. Maximum 8 mg/day. Limit to 12–16 mg/month, at most<br>Prednisone: 20 mg (½ to 1 tablet) every 8–12 h as need. Maximum dose, 40 mg/day. Limit to 80 mg/month, at most | Often very effective therapy for severe, prolonged migraine; dexamethasone and prednisone are very helpful for menstrual migraine<br>The small doses limit side effects, but nausea, anxiety, a "wired" feeling, and insomnia are seen. IV or IM steroids are very effective as well<br>Patients need to be informed of, and accept, the possible adverse events |
| *Ergot* | | | |
| Ergotamine (Ergomar, generics)<br>Ergotamine and caffeine (Cafergot) | Sublingual tablets, suppositories | Varies with preparation<br>Tablets: ½ or 1 tablet once or twice per day as needed | Oldest therapy for migraines. Often effective, but side effects, including nausea and anxiety, are common. Only compounded Cafergot PB is available. The suppositories are more effective than the tablets<br>Rebound headaches are common with overuse of ergots. Use only in younger patients. Ergomar SL tablets are back on the market; contains no caffeine. The Ergomar dose is ½ or 1 tablet once or twice per day as needed |

*ASA* aspirin, *DHE* dihydroergotamine, *GI* gastrointestinal, *IM* intramuscular, *IV* intravenous, *NSAID* nonsteroidal anti-inflammatory drug, *PI* prescribing information

**Table 1.8** Antiemetic medications[a]

| Drug name (brand) | Formulations/dosage | Comments |
|---|---|---|
| Promethazine (Phenergan) | Available as tablets, suppositories, and oral lozenges | Mild but effective for most patients. Very sedating with a low incidence of serious side effects. Used for children and adults. Oral lozenges are formulated by compounding pharmacists |
| Prochlorperazine (Compazine) | IV, tablets, long-acting spansules, and suppositories | Very effective but there is a high incidence of extrapyramidal side effects. Anxiety, sedation, and agitation are common. When given IV, it may stop the migraine pain as well as the nausea |
| Metoclopramide (Reglan) | Oral, IM, and IV; dose: 5–10 mg | Mild, but well tolerated; commonly used prior to IV DHE. Fatigue or anxiety do occur, but usually are not severe. It is pregnancy category B (relatively safe) |
| Trimethobenzamide (Tigan) | Tablets, oral lozenges, and suppositories | Well tolerated, useful in children and adults. Oral lozenges are formulated by compounding pharmacists |
| Ondansetron (Zofran, generic) | Oral tablets and disintegrating tablets; dose: 4 or 8 mg (usually 8 mg every 3–4 h prn) | A very effective antiemetic with few side effects but expensive. It is not sedating. Zofran is extremely useful for patients who need to keep functioning and not be sedated with an antiemetic. It is pregnancy category B (relatively safe) |

*DHE* dihydroergotamine, *IM* intramuscular, *IV* intravenously, *prn* as required

[a] These are commonly prescribed for nausea and other gastrointestinal (GI) symptoms

amine occasionally is useful when administered intramuscularly. At times, patients may have injections for home use (ketorolac, orphenadrine, sumatriptan, diphenhydramine, promethazine, etc.). Transcranial magnetic stimulation (TMS) will soon be available. Patients will have a hand-held device, placed over the occiput, for only a minute. Several quick magnetic pulses are delivered, which are generally very safe. This may be effective for many people. TMS has been around for some time (for depression), in much higher doses, and has been fairly safe and well tolerated.

## *Medication Overuse Headache*

Much is written about MOH, with many patients diagnosed with this condition. Often a patient will be overusing abortive agents but will not be suffering "rebound/withdrawal" headaches (medication overuse, but not MOH). Up until recently, all NSAIDS were lumped under "medications that cause MOH," and this simply is not correct. For some patients, opioids, butalbital, and medications containing a lot of caffeine cause MOH. Triptans are implicated occasionally as well. However, preventives may not be effective for most patients with chronic migraine (daily or near-daily headaches), and they use abortives to help themselves get through the day.

There are more questions in the area of MOH than answers. The pathophysiology of MOH is unclear. Some patients will have MOH from taking two Excedrin daily, while others do not suffer from MOH consuming eight Excedrin per day. When patients are using abortives frequently, we often withdraw them from that abortive, encourage the use of preventives, and attempt to minimize analgesics. However, for many chronic migraine sufferers, preventives are not very effective. For those sufferers, abortives allow them to live with a reasonable quality of life.

## *Preventive Medications*

There are no treatment algorithms to determine which migraine patient should be prescribed preventive headache medication. The choice of who qualifies for medication depends on the patient's age, medical and psychiatric comorbidities, and frequency and severity of the patient's migraine, as well as the patient's preference. Patients have to be willing to take daily medication (many are not). There is no absolute rule that applies to headache treatment. For a patient with two headaches a month that are severe, prolonged, and not relieved by drugs, preventive medicine might be used. On the other hand, for the person who has five headaches a month but can obtain relief from Excedrin or a triptan, preventive medicine may not be optimal.

Comorbidities often determine which preventive medications are used. If a patient has hypertension, a medication for blood pressure will be used. When patients concurrently suffer with anxiety or depression, various antidepressants are utilized to manage the headache and mood disorder. We want to minimize medications and treating two conditions with one medication is ideal.

In using medication, a realistic goal is to decrease the severity of headaches by 40–70 %, not to completely eliminate the headaches. "Clinical meaningful pain relief" usually is around a 30 % improvement. It is wonderful when the headaches are 90 % improved, but the idea is to minimize medication. Most patients need to be willing to settle for moderate improvement. Preventives may take 3–6 weeks to work, and "educated guesswork" often is used to find the best approach for each patient. In the long run, preventive medications are effective for approximately 50 % of patients. The remaining patients try various abortives.

As noted, patients should play an active role in medication choice. Preventive medications should be selected based on the patient's comorbidities, GI system, medication sensitivities, and the like. Fatigue and/or weight gain are major reasons why patients abandon a preventive medication. Headache patients commonly complain of fatigue, and they tend to give up on medications that increase tiredness. A patient's occupation also may guide the caregiver away from certain medications; for example, an accountant may not be able to tolerate the memory problems associated with topiramate.

Side effects are possible with any medication; the patient must be prepared to endure mild side effects to achieve results. Table 1.9 provides a summary of first-line preventive medications.

## *First-Line Preventive Medications for Migraine*

Onobotulinum toxin A has been studied extensively in patients with migraines. Nearly 4 million people have had onobotulinum toxin A injections for headache. Onobotulinum toxin A has been found to significantly improve quality of life and reduce headache impact [7].

Botox is the only onobotulinum toxin A that is FDA-approved for the treatment of chronic migraine. It is relatively safe and only takes a few minutes to inject. One set of injections can decrease headaches for 1–3 months. There also is a cumulative benefit, in which the headaches continue to improve over 1 year of injections. Botox may be safer than many of the medications that are used for headache. Botox does not cause the "annoying" side effects that are commonly encountered with preventives.

The anticonvulsant agents topiramate (Topamax) and valproate acid (Depakote) are FDA-approved as migraine preventives. Topiramate is used to manage migraine, chronic daily headaches, and cluster headache; however, sedation and cognitive side effects, such as confusion or memory problems, may limit its use. Topiramate often decreases appetite, which leads to weight loss; this is unusual among headache preventives. The use of topiramate increases the risk for kidney stones. Bicarbonate levels should be monitored because this agent may cause dose-related metabolic acidosis. This acidosis may lead to "tingling," which sometimes may be counteracted by potassium (in foods or supplements).

**Table 1.9** First-line preventive medications for migraine

| Drug name (brand) | FDA-approved | Formulation | Usual dosage | Comments |
|---|---|---|---|---|
| Onobotulinum toxin A (Botox) | Yes | Injection | Dose: Varies (FDA official dose is 155 units, via 31 injections, every 3 months) | One set of injections can decrease headaches for 1–3 months. Botox is most likely safer than the other medications used for headache. There also is a cumulative benefit, in which the headaches continue to improve over 1 year of Botox therapy |
| *Anticonvulsants* | | | | |
| Topiramate (Topamax) Topiramate ER (Trokendi) | Yes | Oral | Total dose varies from 25 or 50 mg/day up to 400 mg/day | Sedation and cognitive side effects, such as confusion or memory problems, may limit its use; GI upset may occur. Topiramate increases the risk for kidney stones. Bicarbonate levels should be monitored because topiramate may cause dose-related metabolic acidosis |
| Valproic or Divalproex sodium (Depakote) | Yes | Oral | Usual dose: 500–1000 mg/day, in divided doses | Liver function levels need to be monitored in the beginning of treatment. Depakote needs 4–6 weeks to become effective. Side effects include lethargy, GI upset, depression, memory difficulties, weight gain, and alopecia. Depakote should not be used during pregnancy. Available in 125, 250-ER, and 500-ER mg tablets |
| *β-blockers* | | | | |
| Propranolol (Inderal, others) | Yes | Oral | 60–120 mg/day | Side effects include dizziness, insomnia, fatigue, GI upset, respiratory distress, weight gain |
| Metoprolol (Toprol XL) | No | Oral | 25–100 mg/day | Fewer respiratory effects than propranolol |
| Atenolol (Tenormin) | No | Oral | 25–50 mg/day | Fewer respiratory effects than propranolol |
| Nebivolol (Bystolic) | No | Oral | 2.5–10 mg/day | Better tolerated than the other β-blockers with the fewest respiratory effects |

**Table 1.9** (continued)

| Drug name (brand) | FDA-approved | Formulation | Usual dosage | Comments |
|---|---|---|---|---|
| *Tricyclic antidepressants* | | | | |
| Amitriptyline (Elavil, others)<br>Nortriptyline (Pamelor) | No | Oral | Starting dose: 10 mg at bedtime; titrate up to 25–50 mg at night. Maximum dose: 150 mg/day | Effective, inexpensive, and also useful for daily headaches and insomnia. Sedation, weight gain, dry mouth, and constipation are common<br>Nortriptyline, a metabolite of amitriptyline, is somewhat better tolerated (milder) |
| Doxepin (Sinequan) | No | Oral | Starting dose: 10 mg at bedtime; titrate up to 25–50 mg/day. Maximum dose: 150 mg/day | Similar to amitriptyline, with fewer side effects |
| Protriptyline | No | Oral | 5–20 mg/day | Protriptyline is one of the only older antidepressants that does not cause weight gain. However, its anticholinergic side effects are more pronounced. More effective for tension than migraine |
| *NSAIDs*[a] | | | | |
| Naproxen (Aleve, Anaprox, Naprelan, Naprosyn, others) | No | Oral | 500–550 mg/day; maximum dose 1000–1100 mg/day | OTC option. Because of frequent GI side effects, Naproxen is more useful in younger patients, particularly for menstrual migraine<br>With daily NSAIDs, blood tests are needed to monitor liver and kidney function |
| *Calcium channel blocker* | | | | |
| Verapamil | No | Oral | 120 mg/day slow-release tablet, titrate to 240 mg/day | Reasonably effective for migraine. Usually nonsedating; weight gain is uncommon<br>May be combined with other first-line medications, particularly amitriptyline or naproxen<br>With doses higher than 240 mg/day, an ECG needs to be performed. Constipation is common |

*ECG* electrocardiogram, *GI* gastrointestinal, *NSAIDs* nonsteroidal anti-inflammatory drugs, *OTC* over the counter
[a] Other NSAIDs are useful as well

## Natural Supplements and Herbs

Feverfew, Petadolex (butterbur), and magnesium oxide have all proven effective as migraine preventives in double-blind studies. Of these, Petadolex has been the most effective. Petadolex, a purified form of the herb butterbur, is made of extracted plant certified by the German Health Authority. This herb preparation is used commonly in Europe, and has been found to be successful in preventing migraines in several well-designed blind studies. The usual dose is 100 mg/day; many patients require an increase to 150 mg/day (all at once, or in two divided doses). Earlier concerns about carcinogenesis with this family of herbs have decreased with the use of Petadolex. Patients have occasionally experienced GI upset or a bad taste in the mouth, but Petadolex is usually well tolerated. It is prudent to stop it every 3 months or so. Petadolex is available by calling 1-888-301-1084 or through www.petadolex.com or Amazon.com.

Magnesium is a naturally occurring mineral that helps many systems in the body to function, especially the muscles and nerves. It has been shown that magnesium levels in the brain of migraine patients tend to be lower than normal. Magnesium oxide is used as a supplement to maintain adequate magnesium in the body. A dose of 400 or 500 mg/day can be used as a preventive; tablets and powder versions are found in most pharmacies. However, mild GI side effects may limit use. There also are drug interactions that may occur; as always, advise your patients to consult with a physician before taking any supplements.

Feverfew has been demonstrated to be mildly effective in some patients for prevention of migraine headache.

Feverfew can cause a mild increased tendency toward bleeding, and should be discontinued 2 weeks prior to any surgery. The problem with many herbal supplements is quality control. The amount of parthenolide (the active ingredient in feverfew) varies widely from farm to farm; certain farms consistently have better quality herbs than others. It is available in both capsule and liquid forms. The usual dose is two capsules each morning. Patients occasionally will be allergic to feverfew, and it should not be used during pregnancy. Miscellaneous hers/supplements have been used, particularly vitamin B2. CoQ10 and fish oil have also been studied. These occasionally help, but they are less effective than Petadolex (Table 1.10).

## Medications: First Line

As noted, topiramate is an effective migraine preventive. While usually fairly well tolerated, topiramate commonly causes side effects including memory difficulties ("spaciness") and tingling. Topiramate does decrease appetite, leading to weight loss for some patients. This anorexic effect tends to disappear after several months. The usual dose is 50–100 mg daily, but some patients do well on as little as 25 mg/day. The dose may be increased to 300 or 400 mg/day in the absence of significant side effects.

**Table 1.10** Supplements, medicinal herbs, and teas for chronic migraine

| Supplement | Dosage | Uses | Comment |
|---|---|---|---|
| Riboflavin (vitamin B2) | 50–400 mg/day | Prevention | Occasionally helpful, but very mild effect. Higher dose found more effective in reducing number of headaches |
| Magnesium | 200–700 mg/day | Prevention | Magnesium (usually magnesium oxide or citrate) is available in capsule or powder forms. Safe for pregnant women. Not as effective as Petadolex, but occasionally helpful |
| Coenzyme Q10 (CoQ10) | 300–500 mg/day | Prevention | CoQ10 is primarily used to offset side effects of statins, occasionally helpful for migraine. No solid controlled trial data proving efficacy |
| Fish oil(omega-3 fatty acids) | 6000 mg/day | Adjunctive therapy | May represent beneficial adjunctive therapy, but its efficacy as a preventive agent for chronic migraine has not been proven |
| *Medicinal herbs and teas* | | | |
| Botanical name (common name) | Dosage | Uses | Comment |
| Tanacetum parthenium (Feverfew) | 50–143 mg/day | Treatment/prevention | Feverfew is well tolerated, but efficacy is very limited |
| Petasites Petadolex (Butterbur) | 100–150 mg/day | Treatment | Petadolex is the branded, better form of butterbur (Petadolex limits the molecule that is worrisome in butterbur); of the natural supplements, this has the most solid evidence for efficacy<br>Petadolex (Butterbur) is available online at: Petadolex.com or Amazon.com |
| Aromatherapy: lavender/peppermint, and others | Unknown | Symptomatic treatment | Lavender oil (as well as peppermint, and others) applied topically may help reduce sympathetic outflow, reducing pulse and blood pressure, while having a calming effect; aromatherapy is safe and occasionally helpful |
| Salix alba (white willow bark) | 600 mg | Adjunctive therapy | Used for decades, but no true evidence of efficacy |

Valproate, or divalproex sodium (Depakote), is a long-time staple, popular for migraine prevention. It is usually well tolerated in the lower doses used for headaches; however, the generic may not be as effective. Liver functions need to be monitored in the beginning of treatment. Valproate also is one of the primary mood stabilizers for bipolar disorder. Oral Depakote ER (500 mg) is an excellent once-daily, long-acting agent. As with most preventives, valproate needs 4–6 weeks to become effective.

The β-blocker propranolol also is FDA-approved as a preventive agent for migraines. Long-acting oral propranolol (Inderal), for example, is very useful in combination with the tricyclic antidepressant amitriptyline. Dosage begins with the long-acting agent given at 60 mg/day, and usually is kept between 60 and 120 mg/day. Lower doses, such as 20 mg twice per day of propranolol, sometimes are effective. Other β-blockers, such as metoprolol (Toprol XL) and atenolol, also are effective. Some of these are easier to work with than propranolol because they are scored tablets, and metoprolol and atenolol have fewer respiratory effects. Depression may occur. β-blockers are useful for migraine patients with concurrent hypertension, tachycardia, mitral valve prolapse, and panic/anxiety disorders. Bystolic (Nebivolol) is another β-blocker that may be helpful for the prevention of headaches, with the least amount of side effects.

As noted, amitriptyline is an effective, inexpensive agent that is useful for the prevention of daily headaches and insomnia. As a preventive agent, amitriptyline is prescribed at low doses and taken at night. Sedation, weight gain, dry mouth, and constipation are common side effects. Other tricyclic anti-depressants, such as doxepin and protriptyline, can be effective for migraine. Nortriptyline is similar to amitriptyline, with somewhat fewer side effects. These also are used for daily tension-type headaches. Protriptyline is one of the few older antidepressants that does not cause weight gain. However, anticholinergic side effects are increased with protriptyline; protriptyline is more effective for tension headache than for migraine. Although selective serotonin reuptake inhibitors (SSRIs) are used, they are more effective for anxiety and depression than for migraine.

Naproxen is a very useful agent for the treatment of daily headaches, as well as for younger women suffering from menstrual migraine. Naproxen is nonsedating, but it frequently causes GI upset that increases as a person ages. Effective as an abortive, it may be combined with other first-line preventive medications. Other NSAIDs similarly can be used for migraine prevention. As with all anti- inflammatories, GI side effects increase as people age, and, therefore, NSAIDs are used much more frequently in the younger population. Blood tests are needed to monitor liver and kidney function.

## *Second-Line Migraine: Preventive Therapy*

There are a number of second-line migraine treatments (Table 1.11). The antiseizure medication gabapentin has been demonstrated to be useful in migraine and tension headache prophylaxis. In a large study on migraine, doses averaged approximately

**Table 1.11** Second-line migraine preventive therapy[a]

| Drug name (brand) | FDA approved | Formulation | Dosage | Comments |
|---|---|---|---|---|
| Antiseizure medications | | | | |
| Gabapentin (Neurotin, Gralise, others) | No | Oral | Usual dose: 600–2400 mg/day<br>Some patients do well on low doses (100–300 mg/day) | Sedation and dizziness may be a problem; however, gabapentin does not appear to cause end-organ damage, and weight gain is relatively minimal<br>Gabapentin can be used as an adjunct to other first-line preventive medications. Available in 100, 300, 400, 600, and 800 mg doses<br>Gralise is a once-daily, long-acting version of gabapentin |
| Pregabalin (Lyrica) | No | Oral | 25 mg bid to 150 mg tid | Side effects similar to those of gabapentin; possibly causes more weight gain |
| *Muscle relaxants* | | | | |
| Cyclobenzaprine | No | Oral | 5–10 mg/day | Sedation is a common side effect; helpful for sleeping |
| Tizanidine | No | Oral | Usual dose: 2–4 mg every night; patients start with ¼ to ½ tablet. May be increased to 12 mg/day | Safe, nonaddicting agent. Sedation and dry mouth are common<br>Tizanidine may be used on an as-needed basis for milder headaches, or for neck or back pain<br>Available in 2- and 4-mg tablets |
| *Antidepressants* | | | | |
| Desvenlafaxine (Pristiq) | No | Oral | 50–100 mg/day | The antidepressants with dual mechanisms (serotonin and norepinephrine) are more effective for pain and headache than the SSRIs |
| Duloxetine (Cymbalta, generic) | No | Oral | 30–60 mg/day | |
| Venlafaxine (Effexor XR) | No | Oral | 75–225 mg/day | |
| *Natural agent* | | | | |
| Petadolex (purified butterbur) | No | Oral | 100–150 mg/day | Petadolex is very effective; it is a safer form of butterbur. Minimal side effects |

*bid* twice daily, *SSRIs* selective serotonin reuptake inhibitors, *tid* thrice daily

[a] Polypharmacy also is commonly used as second-line treatment of migraine (i.e., amitriptyline with propranolol, or amitriptyline with valproic acid)

2400 mg/day, but lower doses are usually prescribed [8]. Some patients do well with very low doses (200 or 300 mg/day). Sedation and dizziness may be a problem; however, gabapentin does not appear to cause end-organ damage, and weight gain is relatively minimal. Gabapentin can be used as an adjunct to other first-line preventive medications. Pregabalin (Lyrica) has a similar mechanism of action to gabapentin. Pregabalin is fairly safe, but sedation and weight gain often occur.

A safe, nonaddicting muscle relaxant, tizanidine, is useful for migraine and chronic daily headache. Tizanidine may be used on an as-needed basis for milder headaches, or for neck or back pain. Cyclobenzaprine (10 mg) is helpful for sleeping, and it helps some patients with migraine and chronic daily headache. There have been a number of studies on using angiotensin receptor blockers (ARB) and angiotensin-converting enzyme inhibitors (ACEIs) for the prevention of migraine. ARBs are preferred because of minimal side effects.

Examples include losartan (Cozaar), olmesartan (Benicar), and candesartan (Atacand). These may be useful for the patient with hypertension and migraine. Side effects include dizziness, among others, but they are usually well tolerated, with no sedation or weight gain.

Venlafaxine (Effexor XR) is an excellent antidepressant that is occasionally helpful for the prevention of migraine. At lower doses, venlafaxine functions primarily as an SSRI, but at higher doses (100–150 mg), it also increases norepinephrine. In fact, antidepressants with such dual mechanisms (serotonin and norepinephrine) are more effective for pain and headache. Another similar medication is duloxetine (Cymbalta, others), with typical doses being 30–60 mg daily. Duloxetine has several pain indications, but it is probably more effective for moods than for headache. For frontal, severe chronic migraine, sphenopalatine ganglion (SPG) blocks (Marcaine or Lidocaine sprayed up the nose, via a special device) have shown some efficacy, at least in the short term.

## *Polypharmacy*

Polypharmacy is common in migraine prevention. Polypharmacy commonly is employed when significant comorbidities (anxiety, depression, hypertension, etc.) are present. Two first-line medications often are used together and the combination of two preventives can be more effective than a single drug alone [12]. For example, valproic acid (Depakote, or sodium valproate) often is combined with an antidepressant. Amitriptyline may be combined with propranolol (or other β-blockers), particularly if the tachycardia of the amitriptyline needs to be offset by a β-blocker; this combination is commonly used for "mixed" headaches (migraine plus chronic daily headache). NSAIDs may be combined with most of the other first-line preventive medications. Thus, naproxen often is given with amitriptyline, propranolol, or verapamil. Naproxen is employed simultaneously as preventive and abortive medication. Unfortunately, polypharmacy brings the risk of increased side effects.

## *Conclusion*

Migraine is a very common and disabling illness. Outside of medications, it is important for migraineurs to watch their headache triggers and exercise regularly. Physical therapy and/or psychotherapy may be of help—"it takes a village." There is no one algorithm for determining which medication is best for which patient. Each patient is unique, and comorbidities drive where we go with treatment. The goal is to decrease head pain while minimizing medications.

This is an updated version of an article that originally appeared in *Practical Pain Management,* July 2014.

# Chronic Headache Management: Outpatient Strategies

## *A Guide to Treating Chronic Headache Patients*

When we assess patients who seek medical treatment for headache pain, they usually suffer from migraine, tension, or chronic migraine (CM). Only about 5% of patients fall outside of that realm. Cluster headache is another type of primary headache, but cluster headache is relatively uncommon; it is only found in about one out of 250 men and one in 700 women [13]. In contrast, migraine is common; it occurs in 18% of women and 7% of men in the USA. Chronic daily headache (CDH), which is usually CM, often results in a markedly decreased quality of life. We have numerous medications for episodic migraine, but we have less that is effective for CM. The following discussion reviews what we currently know about the various types of headaches, comorbidities, triggers, and treatments.

### Migraine

There are 25–28 million people in the USA with migraine, making it one of the most common of illnesses. Many migraine patients successfully alleviate their headaches with over-the-counter medicines, but most are disabled to one degree or another during the migraine. I look at migraine as an inherited, chronic illness. It is characterized by moderate to severe pain, often unilateral, although it certainly may be bilateral. Migraine is usually accompanied by associated features such as nausea, dizziness, photophobia, sonophobia, or osmophobia. Exacerbation of the headache from bending or other movement is common, as is neck pain. Aura is fairly common; up to 25% of migraineurs experience an aura, but not with every headache. It is common to have prodromal and/or postdromal fatigue and mood changes. Migraine may begin at any age and is surprisingly common in children and adolescents. At least 1% of 6-year-olds and 4% of 10-year-olds suffer from episodic migraine. Until age 12, boys and girls suffer from migraine in equal numbers.

During puberty, the familiar women to men ratio of 3:1 is reached, and that ratio is maintained throughout the rest of life [20].

In diagnosing migraine, it helps to look at consistent triggers—such as menses, weather, and under-sleeping. If weather changes bring on migraine, it is always confusing, since the migraineur is often told (and feels) that they have a sinus headache. To confuse the picture, the OTC sinus meds often help all types of headache. Most sinus headaches turn out to be migraines. There have been several large studies indicating that 95% of people presenting with chronic sinus headaches actually have migraines, not sinus headaches. So one must think "migraine first" regarding pain in the sinus area [2].

## Workup

With a new onset headache—especially in a patient in middle or later life—more extensive workup is needed. This is also true for new neurological symptoms such as numbness, a change in mental status, or visual problems. The patient with CDHs warrants a magnetic resonance imaging (MRI) more often than the patient with sporadic migraines. Children with migraine may not need an MRI. If a 12-year-old presents with two migraines per month since age 6, an MRI is not absolutely necessary. However, when the kids are followed as far as college age, often there will be an incident where they will call and complain of a severe, prolonged headache and usually end up having a scan at some point. Most headache patients should undergo routine hematologic exams, primarily to assess liver and kidney function. Patients are often taking OTC medicines that they do not tell us about. They either do not remember or do not have a sense of how many OTCs they take for pain relief. It is not unusual for headache sufferers to consume eight to ten ibuprofen or Excedrin on a daily basis; the liver and kidneys may be affected.

## Triggers

One of the primary things we can do is educate patients about triggers. Unfortunately, we cannot do very much about certain triggers, but when a patient has a headache every time the weather changes, or the first day of every menstrual period, we might be able to use medicine the day or night before as a preventative. The top triggers tend to be stress (daily hassles), menses, and weather. When they occur simultaneously is when patients get the worst, most prolonged migraines. Of course, missing meals, under- or oversleeping, bright lights, and certain foods also contribute, but the role of foods tends to be overemphasized. People are given a forbidden-food list and told, "Avoid these foods and you won't have headaches," and then they are disappointed. Many books concentrate on diet and foods, but these are low on the list of important triggers. Caffeine, however, is a major trigger. We need to limit the patient's intake, although the limit varies. Some people can consume 800 mg a day of caffeine and not incur rebound headaches or withdrawal. Other people get headaches from a small amount of caffeine in their diet. Caffeine is an adjunct for pain relief as it does help enhance analgesics. Small amounts often help people with their headaches. We have to watch out for the specialty coffeehouse effect. Starbucks coffee has approximately 23 mg of caffeine per ounce. In that oversized cup of Starbucks, you will ingest about 400 mg of caffeine, which is twice the daily maximum recommended. But most home-brewed coffees have manageable doses. Coffees such as Folgers or Hills Brothers have about 150 mg/cup, while instant coffee has half that amount. Tea, if it has caffeine, will generally have 30–60 mg/cup. Cola drinks have 40–60 mg and Mountain Dew has a little more. The new energy drinks may have 200 mg in 12 oz. Watch for accumulated caffeine from these and from OTC medication; each tablet of Excedrin has 65 mg of caffeine, while Anacin has only 33 mg. I attempt to limit a patient's daily caffeine intake to 150 mg—with 200 mg as the maximum [15].

## Psychological Comorbidities

Comorbidities guide what we suggest for headache patients. Psychiatric comorbidities are relatively common in headache patients, primarily due to shared genetic susceptibilities. I tell patients that migraine is an inherited medical problem just like having asthma or diabetes. Similarly, in those with patients suffering anxiety and depression, a genetic tendency can make them susceptible—the same as with diabetes. So, refrain from telling patients that it is all in their heads since they have been told that their entire lives. If we "medicalize" these ailments and remove some of the stigma, patients will allow us to explore more of their psychological conditions. The psychological conditions often drive where we go with treatment.

## Attention-Deficit Disorder

Attention-deficit disorder (ADD) is another important comorbidity. The ADD (in adults) often goes unrecognized and untreated. ADD is common and studies have shown that about 4.7 % of adults have ADD. When someone comes into the office, we are not looking at a just a headache, we are assessing the whole person. If we are able to concurrently manage the comorbidities, the patient will have a better quality of life. The stakes increase with age for untreated ADD. At age 6, kids may not be doing well in school, but by age 26 they are losing their families and their jobs, with a much higher risk for addiction. The risk of addiction for older adolescent boys (8–20-year-olds) having untreated ADD is almost 75 %, usually manifesting as an alcohol problem. If the ADD is treated, the addiction risk decreases to 20–25 % [21]. The stimulants prescribed for ADD often help the headaches as well. Addictions are a comorbidity that complicate the treatment of a refractory patient. Treating pain patients in the face of addiction is complex and often requires a combined psychiatric and medical approach.

### Anxiety

When the comorbidity is anxiety, it is usually generalized anxiety disorder (GAD). OCD is also common, and panic attacks are actually ten times more common in migraine patients than in the general population. Separation anxiety tends to begin early in childhood. We often see social anxiety in high school kids who miss days and even months of school, or are homebound. With these kids, simply prescribing meds is inadequate; we need to recruit psychotherapists in order to address the comorbid anxiety, depression, etc. Whether any adolescent should be homebound because of headaches is controversial. We usually take a nuanced approach to adolescents with severe headaches who miss school. Some do better with online schooling, homebound, or a combination. Certain adolescents require more of a "tough love" approach. If an adolescent has been homebound, it helps to ease them back into school, possibly with a lighter schedule for some period of time.

### Depression

When the comorbidity is depression, it is usually major depression or dysthymia. Of course, many adults with depression are actually bipolar, or fit into the mild bipolar spectrum. Depression is often comorbid in headache patients, most likely due to shared inherited and environmental factors. Unipolar depression, whether it is major depression or dysthymia, is better recognized than bipolar depression. Up to 60 % of adults with chronic depression fit into the bipolar spectrum. It is vital to treat both pain and depression, as they fuel one another. Patients do say, "Of course I am depressed. Wouldn't anyone be with severe headaches?" My answer is, "Headaches do make the depression worse, but many people (60 %) with chronic pain are not depressed. Depression is a separate, biological problem."

### Headache and the Bipolar Spectrum

The relationship between bipolar illness and migraine has not been as well studied as depression and migraine. However, in several studies, the bipolar spectrum has been found at an increased rate in migraineurs. Recent studies confirm that at least 8 % of headache patients also are in the bipolar spectrum. Approximately 4.5 % of the general population fits into the bipolar spectrum [16]. Studies of people with bipolar found that approximately 40 % of bipolar patients also have migraines.

The clinical spectrum of bipolar disorders is an evolving concept. Historically, the *Diagnostic and Statistical Manual of Mental Disorders* (DSM) has inherent biases against independently diagnosing bipolarity, and bipolar II is defined very conservatively in DSM-V. For example, in DSM-V, the important hypomanic reaction to an antidepressant is not included in helping determine bipolarity. The label "bipolar" is unfair and misleading and the associated stigma inhibits diagnosis. We need educational materials aimed at the milder end of the bipolar spectrum.

It is the milder end of the bipolar spectrum that tends to be missed. Look for patients with persistently agitated, angry personalities, with frequent depressions and/or, "too much energy," and having a strong bipolar or depressive family history. Family history also may include substance abuse. Patients may not necessarily have had a clear hypomanic or manic episode. Soft bipolar signs include: early depression (beginning as teens), severe depression, quick onset depression, bipolar reaction to certain meds (up all night, thoughts racing, etc.), agitated and angry depression, very high anxiety and mood swings, poor response to medication, and moody personality. Sleep disorders are commonly seen. Cyclical depression, "for no reason," along with high anxiety is common for bipolar depression. The therapeutic implications for recognizing bipolarity are enormous. These patients tend to bounce from antidepressant to antidepressant with predictably poor results. Mood stabilizers—lithium, lamotrigine, and atypicals such as quetiapine and aripiprazole—are much more effective.

### Personality Disorders

It is crucial to recognize personality disorders (PDs) within your practice. Approximately 10% of people have strong features of a PD. Approximately 5% of migraineurs have one of the more severe PDs: borderline, narcissistic, antisocial, and paranoid. There are a number of PDs, some of which are more dangerous and difficult to deal with than others. In general, characteristics of PDs include: lack of insight; poor response to psychotherapy or other therapeutic interventions; difficulty with attachments and trust; a sense of entitlement; the creation of a great deal of chaos and distress in family, friends, and coworkers; etc.

PDs have a wide range of severity, from mild to very severe. These individuals often flip between victim, rescuer, and persecutor. When they turn persecutor, they can be dangerous to the person they have their sights set on. PD patients often create chaos and drama, and comorbid substance abuse is common. They also bring chaos and drama to the medical clinic. The more difficult PDs include paranoid, antisocial, borderline, and narcissistic behaviors. In general, therapy helps people with PDs only over long periods of time. Dialectical therapy is usually preferred for those with a PD. Seeing a therapist for 5–7 years may help to some degree. However, our goals and expectations are limited. The concept of plasticity of the brain is very important, as some people do improve naturally over time. One study of borderline PD in adolescents indicated that, by age 30, one third of the subjects no longer had borderline PD. Many people do not fit neatly into any of these categories, but have features of two or three PD types. Failure to identify those with PDs leads to increased risk for the provider and the patient. The small percentage of patients with moderate-to-severe PDs in a typical practice are the ones who create the majority of the drama, as well as legal and regulatory problems for the treating physicians [18].

## Medical Comorbidities

As far as medical comorbidities in headache patients, the GI system is a common site—particularly irritable bowel syndrome (IBS). Most of one's serotonin is in the gut, and certain medicines that help IBS increase or decrease serotonin. IBS is frequently encountered in migraine patients, and very often we are trying to use medicines that help the GI symptoms as well as the headache. It is much easier to help patients who primarily have diarrhea since some of our medicines, such as the older tricyclics, slow the gut transit time. Constipation, on the other hand, is tougher to ameliorate. Some other comorbidities include hypertension, insomnia, fibromyalgia (or chronic pain syndrome), and fatigue.

Central sensitization syndromes include, among others: CM, IBS, fibromyalgia, and chronic pelvic pain. Many people suffer from more than one of these illnesses, which complicates the treatment. Comorbidities drive where we go with chronic pain patients.

### Hypertension

A number of the antihypertensives do diminish migraine. Most β-blockers will help, as will the calcium channel blockers. More recently, the ARBs have been utilized.

### Insomnia

Sleep disorders are frequently encountered with headache patients. Insomnia is common, but the available treatments are not ideal. Of course, we should institute sleep rules and behavioral treatments. For patients with comorbid insomnia and headache, sedating tricyclic antidepressants may be of benefit. Also, certain muscle relaxants, such as tizanadine or cyclobenzaprine, may help both conditions. Of course, we need more effective insomnia meds.

### Fibromyalgia (or Chronic Pain Syndrome)

We do have a few drugs that are indicated for fibromyalgia. Many people with fibromyalgia also have CDHs and insomnia. These groups overlap, not only with the pain but the psychological comorbidities as well. Fibromyalgia patients share the allodynia commonly felt by headache patients. A number of medicines are used for both headache and fibromyalgia, such as tricyclics and muscle relaxants.

### Fatigue

If you ask large groups of headache or migraine patients what their biggest problem is other than headache pain, it tends to be excessive daytime sleepiness. Fatigue is such a prevalent problem that we do not want to add medicines that fatigue people even more. There are no algorithms for headache patients since everyone is different. For example, suppose a woman comes in who is 45 years old and 25 lb overweight and is always tired. We do not want to prescribe amitriptyline or valproate, medicines that are going to make her more tired and gain more weight. Some medicines do not exacerbate fatigue, such as protriptyline (Vivactil) or ARBs, and, occasionally, we will use small doses of stimulants. Modafinil (Provigil) or Nuvigil may offset the fatigue, but do not help headaches. These are expensive medications. However, modafinil or Nuvigil do improve quality of life for many headache patients.

## Outside of Medicine

It does take a village to treat a severe pain patient. We want to seek treatments outside of the pharmacy. We need to promote active coping. We must have other modalities involved. Pharmacotherapy may be important, but certainly we want to try everything else, whether it is physical therapy, yoga, biofeedback, etc. Psychotherapy is often important and I strongly recommend it as part of treatment. However, whether it is because of money or time, most people will not see a therapist. Cognitive-behavioral therapy is the usual approach, but with PDs one must take more of a dialectical tack. It is important to identify the best therapists in your area, as the skill levels of psychotherapists vary widely.

### Acceptance

Acceptance of the pain as an illness is a very important concept. There are actually scales that measure acceptance. The road to acceptance of a chronic illness is often littered with many wrong turns along the way, looking for miracle cures. When people accept that they have a chronic illness, which may be managed but not cured, the inner angst decreases remarkably. Acceptance does not mean that patients are resigned to a lifetime of severe pain, it simply leads to management, not false hope.

### Biofeedback

Biofeedback is a very useful tool. I think that the providers who have been trained in the past 5 or 10 years often do a better job with biofeedback. The home-based therapies involving relaxation techniques—where patients are taught by just giving them a booklet and tapes—can help but a good biofeedback therapist is much more effective. When it is done well, biofeedback promotes an internal locus of control and helps promote self-efficacy. Exercise and yoga can have similar effects. We want people to feel that they can engender a positive outcome in their illness by doing something other than taking a pill Meditation may also help.

### Resilience

Resilience is an interesting concept. Resilience involves the early life experiences as well as genetics. In looking at resilience in individuals, the serotonin transporter gene is crucial. There are two arms on the gene, which can be either short or long. If a person has two long arms on the serotonin transporter gene, it turns out that he is going to be a lot more resilient. His childhood may be unhappy, but when the person has two long arms on the gene, he usually turns out very well. If the patient has an abusive childhood, and he has two short arms on the serotonin transporter gene, it is almost a certainty that he is going to have major problems in life, possibly borderline PD, or some other major psychiatric problem. So resilience is very important in terms of who can cope despite severe headaches, and who ends up disabled.

### Exercise

We try to have patients average 15 or 20 min of any exercise. This includes light walking, treadmill, bike, elliptical, yoga, Pilates, etc. Even 5 or 10 min twice a day is sufficient. The idea with many chronic pain sufferers is to encourage any exercise. The old mantra of "you have to go to the gym, work out for an hour, get your heart rate up yada yada" actually has inhibited people from doing at least some exercise. Many headache patients suffer from "exercise-induced headaches." The smoother, slower types of exercise minimize the headaches.

## Disability and Catastrophizing

One might think that the pain level is the major predictor of disability. It has been shown, in well-done studies, that other factors are probably more important. Catastrophizing is one of these factors. For example, a patient who seems to think his headache is always a 14 on a scale of 1–10. Part of my job is to turn down the volume and limit the drama. We can talk to people about catastrophizing and work on the fear that underlies it. Catastrophizing by proxy also happens, where a parent thinks his child has the worst headaches on the planet and even says, "Have you ever seen such bad headaches in a kid before?" Fear of pain also plays a role in disability. Some people have more fear and anticipation of pain than others and, as with catastrophizing, fear of pain may be lessened through psychotherapy.

### Neck and Occipital Pain

Physical therapy can be very helpful when there is associated pain in the neck and shoulders. At least half of headache patients have neck pain, particularly with their migraines. I often advocate physical therapy for the neck pain, posterior headaches, and jaw pain (many headache patients clench and brut). There are better medical doctors than others and there are better physical therapists than others. It is worthwhile to establish a relationship with the best "headache/neck pain" physical therapists in your area. Occipital pain may be originating in the cervical region; blocks or injections may help.

### Dental, Massage, Acupuncture

Dental consultations may be beneficial for those who clench their jaw, and certainly if they are bruxing. For the associated clenching, bite splints may help, along with physical therapy. Massage can benefit a wide range of patients, but the benefits often are short-lasting. It has been difficult to prove in studies that acupuncture is more effective than sham treatment. After examining more than 500 randomized controlled trials of acupuncture for various conditions, nothing definite can be concluded as far as efficacy [5]. I think, with many pain studies, the outcome of the study can be predicted from how robust the placebo response is. Unfortunately, with acupuncture studies, when the sham acupuncture is performed along with the real acupuncture, there is going to be a robust placebo response. It has been difficult to prove efficacy over placebo. But, there are patients who do very well with acupuncture. Acupuncturists are another one of the "villagers" whom we recruit to help take care of pain patients.

### Medications: Abortives

Most people with migraines do not need preventive medicines, particularly when they do not have comorbidities or not enough headaches. There is no good algorithm that applies to headache treatment. How many headaches a month are too many? With two headaches a month that are severe and prolonged and are not relieved by drugs, we might use preventive medicine. For another person with five headaches a month, who can take an Excedrin or a triptan and obtain relief, we may choose not to use preventive medicine, because all meds have their possible side effects.

For abortives, there are many choices among the triptans. Injections of sumatriptan are probably the most effective. The generic sumatriptan injections are available in several forms: an EpiPen, prefilled syringes, and the generic for the Stat Dose system. All of the triptans are effective, but they each have different clinical characteristics. The generic tablets include: sumatriptan, rizatriptan, naratriptan, and zolmitriptan. Sumatriptan, rizatriptan, zolmitriptan, and Relpax have slightly better efficacy than naratriptan and Frova. Naratriptan and Frova are slow-onset, longer-acting meds. The triptan nasal sprays, particularly Zomig, are fast acting. Side effects of tingling and pressure may initially occur with the triptans. Since 1992, we have had more than 200 million people treated with the triptans. Safety has been well established. We have become more comfortable using triptans in higher-risk populations. If one triptan is ineffective, I usually will try one or two other triptans before giving up on the class. During pregnancy, particularly after the first trimester, triptans may be safer than many of the other migraine medications. The 16-year sumatriptan/naratriptan pregnancy registry demonstrated the relative safety during pregnancy. We use triptans cautiously, with informed consent.

Other than the triptans, most patients have tried over-the-counter products (ibuprofen, naproxen, aspirin, and caffeine combinations). Aspirin and metoclopramide combined may help. Prodrin is an interesting product, with a combination of a small amount (20 mg) of caffeine, acetaminophen, and a mild vasoconstrictor. For those intermediate headaches a reasonable choice, and is not addicting. Prodrin is similar to Midrin (generic Midrin is available), without the sedative in Midrin.

Transcranial magnetic stimulation (TMS) is a safe, noninvasive abortive treatment. Patients may use the stimulator at home; it only takes a few minutes. Over the coming few years, TMS will achieve a larger role as an abortive. There is a solid track record of TMS for depression, and it appears to be safe; for depression, thousands of pulses are given; for headache, only two pulses or so.

DHE is probably underutilized. DHE nasal spray (Migranal: generic available) is safe, but is not always effective. Migranal often leads to severe nasal congestion. DHE injections are much more effective, but are expensive, and often are not available. There is an inhaled version of DHE in the works, and should be available soon. It appears as if the inhaled DHE works better than the nasal spray, but not quite as effective as the injections. Since 1945, when DHE was introduced, there have been relatively few severe side effects reported. An inhaled version of DHE should be available soon. DHE is primarily a venoconstrictor, so it actually safer than other ergotamines, which are arterial constrictors [11].

Antiemetics are important adjuncts for those with nausea. Ondansetron lets people get on with their day without sedation. We also use the other antiemetics, such as metoclopramide or prochlorperazine, which are somewhat sedating. The goal is to keep people out of the emergency room (ER), and the antiemetics help in this regard. I do use opioids and butalbital in selected patients. We limit their use, but nine out of ten patients do not overuse them. It is the 10% who create problems. Butalbital compounds are controversial, and are not used in Europe. Butalbital does result in rebound headaches more than with simple analgesics. Opioid and butalbital use in the headache patient has been found to be one source of transformation from episodic headache into daily pain.

Occasionally, we will use injectable opioids. Alternatively, as a last resort, other parenteral opioids may be of use. These include butorphanol nasal spray, or various forms of fentanyl oral preparations. Butorphanol and fentanyl are highly addicting, and frequently cause side effects. The quicker-onset medicines do tend to be overused, and there are more withdrawal symptoms. These parenteral opioids should be used very sparingly in carefully selected patients. As a last resort, when sedation is needed, we will occasionally use meds off-label, such as quetiapine (Seroquel), or benzodiazepines. When nothing works for refractory headaches, particularly for prolonged menstrual migraines, we do use corticosteroids, but in limited amounts. It is important to minimize the cortisone dose. We use dexamethasone, 4 mg, ½ or 1 every 12 h "as needed"; or prednisone, 20 mg, ½ or 1 every 12 h "as needed." The cortisone "dose packs" deliver a higher dose than is usually necessary. I would usually limit these to three or four tablets a month, at most.

## CM Meds

When it comes to preventives, each person is unique. While comorbidities guide how we proceed, patient preferences are also important. Patients have to be willing to put up with possible side effects. We tend to use more preventives in people with CDH (which is usually CM) than in semimonthly migraines. CM is basically defined as headaches occurring at least 15 days per month, of which at least eight fulfill probable migraine. About 3 % of people, in almost every country that has been assessed, have CDH, or frequent headaches. CM greatly decreases one's quality of life. It is a major problem, it is difficult to treat, and most analgesic overuse stems from CM. The severity of the daily headache is important. Some people will say, "My daily headaches don't bother me, they're mild; it's the severe migraines that are important." Other people say, "It's these daily headaches that are the problem, the moderate or severe migraines are easily taken care of." We aim our preventive meds at the predominant, more severe type of headache. With chronic headache, we need to limit the drugs prescribed as abortives. If patients are taking OTC medications and need to take more than two a day, we must consider daily preventive medicine. We might consider NSAIDs or Prodrin, neither of which are addicting. Triptans may be utilized, but overuse may lead to rebound. Tramadol is a mild opioid. Tramadol ER may be useful if patients can limit use to 200 mg/day, or less. Any medication used abortively for CDH should be strictly limited to two per day.

## Abortives and Rebound Headache (Medication Overuse Headache)

The abortives for CM are basically the same as for episodic migraine. We do not want to use triptans on a daily basis, except in unusual circumstances. Rebound headache is always a consideration and is a remarkably complex subject. The term medication overuse headache has been overused. Many patients are labeled as having medication overuse headache, when in fact they simply have frequent migraines. The major question with rebound headache is which drugs, and how much of the drug, will trigger rebound. It appears that the butalbital and opioid meds, and the high caffeine drugs—such as Excedrin—may be more likely to cause rebound. It appears that in selected patients, NSAIDs may contribute to rebound, but in general they do not.

### Preventives: Long-Term Results

The goal with preventives is to help reduce the headache by 25–75 %. If patients believe that their headaches are going to be completely cured, they may return and state, "The medicines are not working because I still have some migraines." They may be 50 % improved, which is often the best that can be achieved. Headache diaries (or apps, such as ChronicPainTracker) may help, but we also need to convey realistic goals to the patient. In my experience, only 50 % of people do well for the long-term on preventives. I have done two studies looking at usage over a year's time, with a total of nearly 800 patients on preventives. Only 46 % found any preventive that they could tolerate, and that remained effective for at least 9 months [19]. The remainder discontinued preventives for various reasons. We desperately need more effective preventives, with less side effects.

### Natural Remedies

Natural remedies may help, without the common side effects seen with our usual preventives. Petadolex is an improved form of the herb butterbur, where the molecule that we worry about in butterbur is limited. Petadolex is effective, and held up well in randomized controlled trials. It was popular in a number of countries—for instance, in Germany where Petadolex was the number one preventive. I find it is more effective than feverfew, etc. In my years of experience with Petadolex, very few side effects have been reported. Occasionally, there is an upset stomach or a bad taste in the mouth. There is still a concern with carcinogenic properties, particularly with the parent compound of butterbur. We stop the Petadolex periodically for 1–2 months. Most people in the USA order Petadolex directly from the company (1–888-301–1084, Petadolex.com), or from Amazon. We also use magnesium oxide or citrate, 400–600 mg daily. I believe that the Petadolex and magnesium are the most consistently helpful of the natural supplements. Feverfew lags behind as far as efficacy, but it is fairly safe. I have not found vitamin B-2 (200–400 mg daily) to be very helpful in the long term, but occasionally it has been effective.

### Tricyclics

Tricyclics remain a mainstay of headache treatment. With amitriptyline and nortriptyline, we do encounter weight gain, dry mouth, and constipation, but we use small-to-medium doses for most patients. I will start a patient on 5 mg (half of a 10 mg tablet of amitriptyline). The cost of medicine has increased but the generic tricyclics are very inexpensive. Some people remain on 10 mg or 20 mg/day of amitriptyline for years, doing very well. Amitriptyline is metabolized into nortriptyline; nortriptyline has fewer side effects. Protriptyline is one of the only tricyclics that does not cause weight gain, but it may cause anticholinergic side effects. With protriptyline, patients experience dry mouth and constipation, but there is minimal sedation, without the weight gain.

### Anticonvulsants

The primary anticonvulsants have been topiramate and sodium valproate (Topamax®, topiramate ER, generic topiramate, and Depakote® (generic available)). These are indicated for migraine. With topiramate, memory difficulties and mental fog are common. Depression or anxiety may occur as well. As the dose is increased, tingling of the extremities may be present due to carbonic anhydrase effects. Headache patients often quit the preventives due to annoying side effects, and so it is crucial to keep the dosage to a minimum. We try to start low and build up the dose. With topiramate, I will slowly increase to 50 mg and then, if needed, up to 100 mg; many patients do well on 25 or 50 mg. The generic topiramate ER is longer acting. While, the average dose of 500–1000 mg of sodium valproate (Depakote®) may lead to weight gain, topiramate may enhance weight loss. Unfortunately, the anorexic effects of topiramate do wane over a number of months. However, with sodium valproate, we see the weight gain often leading to discontinuation. Of course, we do never want a patient to become pregnant while on sodium valproate. We will start with 250 mg of sodium valproate and move up very slowly. Many other anticonvulsants have been used for headache, without solid studies to back up use. Oxcarbazepine (Trileptal®) has failed in several headache studies, though it probably is an effective mood stabilizer for some patients. Zonisamide (Zonegran®) has been used; it is a once-a-day, longer-acting, relatively safe anticonvulsant. Fatigue is the primary side effect. Zonisamide is usually started at 25 mg at night, and slowly titrated up to 100 mg. Zonisamide does not cause weight gain. Gabapentin has been widely utilized, as has pregabalin (Lyrica), but evidence is lacking for positive efficacy.

### Antihypertensives and Muscle Relaxants

The antihypertensive meds are useful as preventives: β-blockers and calcium channel blockers are the ones most commonly prescribed. There have been studies on the angiotensin renin blockers (ARBs). We encounter fewer side effects with ARBs. Tiredness and weight gain are major problems in migraineurs, and β-blockers exacerbate fatigue and weight gain. So I often use one of the ARBs: Candesartan (Atacand) is the primary ARB that's been studied, but others have been utilized. Muscle relaxants certainly may help the associated neck pain and may aid sleeping. Tizanidine is nonaddicting and is fairly safe, but we use it mostly at night due to the sedation. Cyclobenzaprine is inexpensive, and the tablets can be cut in half. Sedation is often a problem with these muscle relaxants.

## Refractory Headache: Botulinum Toxin Type A

Onabotulinumtoxin A (Botox) is Food and Drug Administration (FDA) indicated for CM (the only FDA-indicated preventive for CM). It has been daunting to prove that it works better than placebo, as the placebo response has been high in several of the Botox studies. In one major study, the placebo response was only about 21 %, but in others, it has been higher. Placebo response in migraine preventive studies, across all trials, averages about 20–23 %. For unknown reasons, the placebo response is lower in North America, by about 5 %, than in Europe [1]. The placebo response also differs among countries in Europe. In a number of Botox studies, the placebo response led to failure in achieving the primary endpoint, but the Preempt Botox study in North America was positive [10]. Many patients do find that it works well for 10–14 weeks. They use considerably less medicine in the two to three months post-Botox, and they can feel the effects wearing off at 2.5–3.5 months. We now have had many years (since 1996) of Botox use for migraine, and one could make a strong case that it is probably safer than most of the other drugs that we use, with fewer side effects. The mechanism for why it works could be due to calcitonin gene-related peptide (CGRP) antagonism, or a similar anti-inflammatory effect. The usual dose, the FDA-indicated dose, is 155 units, distributed about the head in 31 injections. Botox usually takes 5 days to 2 weeks to become effective. There is evidence that Botox becomes more effective over time. Money is the primary concern with the use of Botox, but many insurances, and Medicare, provide reasonable coverage.

## Long-Acting Opioids for Refractory Headache

What to do when nothing works? For refractory patients, long-acting opioids are a possibility. I previously assessed, over a period of 6 years, patients who used long-acting opioids [17]. We looked at comorbidities and predictors of overuse. The people who tend to overuse long-acting opioids are those who previously overused short-acting opioids. If they abused hydrocodone, they tended to overuse the long-acting Morphine ER (Kadian®), Oxycontin®, or methadone. I have not encountered many cases of pseudoaddiction. As a result, I am reluctant to prescribe the long-acting opioids to those individuals who previously overused the short-acting opioids.

We also assessed bipolar, ADD, depression and anxiety, and PDs. The other predictor for overuse of opioids is the presence of a PD. If people have more than a mild PD, opioids are not a good choice. However, for the right person, these drugs can be lifesavers, improving quality of life and functioning. The ideal candidate for long-acting opioids is one who: did well on short-acting opioids (without overuse), has no PD, is greater than 30 years of age, and does not develop tolerance to the analgesic effects. When nothing else works, taking long-acting morphine, buprenorphine, oxycodone, methadone, or hydrocodone in low doses may be effective. Not every doctor should prescribe opioids; there needs to be careful patient selection and good psychiatric screening, and solid documentation with each visit. For certain select patients, opioids will lead to improved functioning, and if lucky they will not develop tolerance to the analgesic effects. Older patients, whose brains cannot do the "neuronal gymnastics" needed to become tolerant, may do well on the same low dose for many years. For a small group of refractory patients, the long-acting opioids may be worthwhile.

### Frequent Triptans: Sumatriptan, Rizatriptan, etc.

There are many patients taking daily, or near-daily, triptans. Some are experiencing rebound headaches from the triptans, but they say, "If I don't take my triptan, I have a severe headache and need to take 6 to 10 Excedrin!" We need more studies of people who need frequent triptans. I published one study of 100 patients, where we did cardiac echocardiograms and electrocardiograms (ECGs). In this particular study, no long-term adverse effects were found. The patients averaged near-daily triptans for almost 4 years [14]. I do not encourage frequent use, but many people do lapse into it. The physician must attempt to withdraw the person from frequent triptans for a period of time, and assess for MOH. There are CM sufferers who do well only with the triptans.

### Refractory Patients: Stimulants

A case can be made for utilizing stimulants in selected patients. They may help with fatigue, concentration, and moods. In the right person, low doses of stimulants are remarkably useful. For some people, stimulants not only improve the quality of life, they also help alleviate the headache pain. There have been several stimulant studies in daily headache patients; I believe that stimulants are underutilized.

### Refractory Patients: Monoamine Oxidase Inhibitors

Monoamine oxidase inhibitors (MAOIs) have fallen out of favor, but occasionally they provide excellent relief for selected patients. Phenelzine is the usual MAOI for headache patients. Low doses are utilized, 15–45 mg daily; if used all at night, food interactions are minimized. For those with refractory headache and comorbid unipolar depression, MAOIs should be considered. Of course, drug interactions and dietary restrictions limit use.

### Refractory Patients: Occipital Stimulators, TMS, and SPG Blocks

In refractory patients, the use of an occipital stimulator is controversial. The stimulator help for a period of time, but it is difficult to anchor the leads, and migration away from the occipital nerve often occurs. Many patients require another surgery for a variety of reasons. Long-term efficacy and safety is questionable. TMS is much easier and is noninvasive, patients may do this at home, and will have a larger role in the next several years. SPG blocks, given once or twice weekly for several weeks, are safe and sometimes effective for daily frontal CM. The three devices on the market are: SphenoCath, Tianx360, and the AllevioSPG. Each device has its pluses and minuses. The SPG block is done in the office, is fairly quick, but there are a limited number of physicians who do this block.

### Patent Foramen Ovale and Migraines

The jury is still out on the issue of patent foramen ovale (PFO; the hole in the heart that may contribute to headache). One recent trial did not reach its primary endpoint but the endpoint chosen was a very difficult one [9]. Several trials are still in progress, seeking to assess whether closure of a PFO will decrease migraines. It is likely that, in a select group of migraineurs with a sizable PFO, closure will significantly decrease the headache frequency.

### Conclusion

Comorbidities often drive where we go with headache patients. It "takes a village" to help a severe headache or pain patient. We consider involving psychotherapists and physical therapists, among others. We want to achieve a balance between headaches and medication, and try to minimize drug usage. Most patients do well with the usual ministrations, but for the refractory patient we need to consider other approaches. When used appropriately, some of these "out of the box" therapies are the key to restoring a patient's quality of life. Note: This is an updated version of an article that originally appeared in *Practical Pain Management,* vol 8, Nov 2008.

## Clinical Pearls for Treating Headache Patients

These clinical tips for headache treatment run the gamut from medication and patient perception to broader health issues and strategies/procedures.

This is the latest in our series of clinical pearls for practical headache treatment. Headache patients often have complex medical and psychological issues, and these pearls hope to offer concise tidbits and suggestions regarding medications, how patients may perceive their condition, broader health options available, and strategies and protocols that may be beneficial.

## *Medication*

- Start with low doses of medication, particularly with antidepressants and other preventives. Headache patients tend to be fairly somatic, and there is no need to push medicine very quickly.
- Stick with preventive medications for at least 4 weeks (or longer). If we abandon them too soon, we may not see the beneficial effect. However, few patients are willing to wait months for positive benefits from a medication.
- Consider newer abortive medications, such as Cambia (powdered diclofenac potassium; not sodium: The sodium version, such as Voltaren, will not work as a powder). Cambia, used in water or apple juice, achieves detectable blood levels in as little as 10 min. Prodrin (isometheptene/acetaminophen/caffeine) is a newer version of Midrin (isometheptene/dichloralphenazone/acetaminophen) with no sedative (Prodrin eliminates the dichloralphenazone) or caffeine. An inhaled version of dihydroergotamine (DHE) is expected to be approved by the Food and Drug Administration (FDA) and will be a better product than Migranal nasal spray, but not quite as effective as injections of DHE. Sphenopalatine ganglion (SPG) blocks, done in office, are usually considered treatments to stop a cycle of frontal migraines (or clusters), but may work abortively for one severe headache.
- Consider natural alternatives that work, such as Petadolex, the butterbur derivative. Petadolex is a highly regulated "adulterated herb," and it had been the No. 1 preventive in Germany. I feel Petadolex is relatively safe, has a long successful track record, and is almost as effective as our mainstream preventives. We do stop the Petadolex for a month every so often. Magnesium and vitamin B2 are also used, but are not as effective as Petadolex. Turmeric and ginger may be an alternative for some patients.
- OnabotulinumtoxinA (Botox) should be considered early in the course of treatment. Botox is now FDA approved for chronic migraine (15 or more days per month). Botox has proven to be safe and effective (almost 60 % of patients experience meaningful relief for 3 months). The cost is a concern. Botox is twice as effective as our usual daily preventive drugs, without the side effects.
- Previous sensitivities and allergies to medications often determine where we go with medications. If the patient has had severe reactions to two SSRIs, a third is not a good choice. However, those reactions may not be readily apparent in the chart. If they are extremely fatigued on one β-blocker, a second will probably not work for the long term.
- Weight gain is a major issue. Even though a drug may be more effective, choosing one that avoids weight gain (in those prone to it) is more likely to lead to long-term success. Fatigue is another major reason for patients abandoning a preventive medication. Headache patients commonly complain of fatigue. Many of our preventives (amitriptyline, β-blockers, valproate, etc.) may add to weight gain and/or fatigue.
- While most patients are honest about analgesic use, some are embarrassed to tell us how much they are utilizing. Between over-the-counter analgesics and herbal

preparations, many patients are consuming larger quantities of medications than we realize. That is one reason to regularly test liver and kidney functions (blood tests).

- Do not confuse addiction with dependency. When treating chronic daily headache, dependency has to be accepted. Dependency is acceptable, while addiction is not.
- When using opioids, you must be willing to say no and set limits. Refrain from using opioids in younger patients, so as to avoid "opioid hyperalgesia." Once younger people are on frequent opioids for a period of time, they may be "sensitized," and we may have little choice but to use opioids.
- Heed red flags in your patients on opioids. While pervasive behaviors help to determine addiction, even one red flag early in treatment should be seriously considered. For instance: You see a new patient, begin Tylenol #3 (codeine/acetaminophen), and receive a call 4 days later from the patient stating, "I got the generic, but the regular works better. Can you call some in?" Or, "I left my codeine in the hotel room"…….If you discover the urine tox screen is abnormal, or that the patient is receiving addicting meds from other doctors, these must be addressed, not ignored.
- Using a medication to establish a diagnosis may not be accurate. For instance, DHE and triptans have also been effective for relieving the pain of nonaneurysmal subarachnoid hemorrhage and tumors.
- What to do when nothing works: Before "giving up" on a patient with severe, refractive chronic daily headache, consider "end of the line" strategies such as daily triptans in limited amounts, Botox injections, monoamine oxidase inhibitors, daily long-acting opioids, stimulants, or a combination of approaches. SPG blocks for frontal pain, using one of the newer devices (SphenoCath or Tx360), along with occipital injections for posterior pain, may help.

## *Patient Perceptions*

- Legitimize the headache problem as a physical illness. Statements such as, "headaches are just like asthma, diabetes, or hypertension: a physical medical condition," go a long way toward establishing trust between the patient and physician. When we mention that it is a medical condition—primarily inherited—and that there is too little serotonin in the brain in people with headaches, patients respond exceedingly well. Once we have established this, the patients are much more amenable to addressing anxiety, depression, etc., with therapy or other means. However, if we focus on the patient's stress, anxiety, depression, and psychological comorbidities first, they are often turned off to the physician unless we also state that we are treating the headaches as a legitimate medical illness.
- When we place patients on antidepressants, we need to make it clear that we are trying to directly help their headache by increasing serotonin. We also state that

we certainly hope this helps anxiety, depression, etc. Patients are often confused as to the reason why they are given an antidepressant. It helps if we make it clear that we are not trying to treat their headache by treating depression, but rather trying to adjust serotonin levels. If the patient does report that the antidepressant made them feel "wired, racy, I was up all night", consider the soft end of the bipolar spectrum.

- We must try to achieve a balance between medication and headache; we tell the patients that we are trying to improve the headaches by 50–90 %, while minimizing medications. Many refractory patients are more than willing to accept 25 % relief.
- Many patients are frustrated by the lack of efficacy and/or side effects of daily preventives. Tell them that only 50 % of patients (at most) achieve long-term relief with preventives. This helps them to realize they are in a big boat, and that it is not their fault. Our current daily preventives often become ineffective over time, or patients cannot tolerate them.
- Patients with chronic daily headache may view the headache situation in black and white terms. They will come back for a return visit and state, "Well, I still have a headache every day." They need to accept that if we have gone from moderate-to-severe headaches (7 on a scale of 1–10) to mild-to-moderate (4 on a scale of 1–10), then the situation is improved and we should not change all the medication. If the patients keep a headache chart or calendar, this may help. Patients need to be willing to accept 50–90 % improvement in frequency and/or severity of headaches.
- Being aware that there are cultural and ethnic differences in the perception and experience of pain can aid treatment.
- Pain patients are often desperate and search the Internet for a cure or seek alternative practitioners. We should not castigate them for doing so; they are just looking for answers.
- Catastrophizing greatly inhibits patients from improving. Work with your patient on decreasing the level of catastrophizing and histrionics. This will improve the pain level and associated anxiety.
- When patients feel they can actively help their headaches ("self-efficacy") through medication, biofeedback, or other means, it improves their sense of well being. Whether by taking a medication, watching triggers, exercising, or doing yoga, etc., increasing "self-efficacy" enhances outcomes.
- Acceptance of their chronic illness (headache) is a helpful state of mind for patients to achieve. Acceptance is different from resignation. Acceptance helps to ease anxiety ("Isn't there a cure? These must be curable"). The road to acceptance may take years, and involve many doctors and alternatives. Lack of acceptance leads to frustration, and wasted time and money seeking the miracle "aha moment" cure. Lack of acceptance "by proxy" also occurs, as parents of children with headaches sometimes refuse to believe that kids can have daily headaches. They also will seek sudden "miracle" cures that almost never happen. The physician and psychotherapist can work on increasing acceptance.

## *Broader Health*

- It can "take a village to help a person with severe pain." Do not try to do it all by yourself; get other villagers involved, including psychotherapy, massage, physical therapy, pain specialists, acupuncture, etc. Direct the patient to whichever of these other professionals is appropriate.
- In choosing preventives, look at comorbidities, particularly anxiety, depression, insomnia, gastritis, gastroesophageal reflux disease, blood sugar, constipation, hypertension, asthma, and sensitivities or allergies to other drugs. These often determine which way to proceed with medication.
- Central sensitization is an important phenomenon that occurs in chronic headache, peripheral neuropathy, and probably also in irritable bowel syndrome (IBS) and fibromyalgia. Once this occurs, treatment is difficult.
- Virtually all patients should be on vitamin D, usually at least 2000 units. Vitamin D is almost "the last man standing" among supplements. Vitamin D helps skin and bones, prevents certain types of cancers, and may help to minimize depression and pain. Multivitamins have more negatives than positives for many patients, and the same is true for antioxidants. Both multivitamins and antioxidants have been associated with increased cancer rates. Even omega-3 fish oil capsules have failed to provide positive benefit in most studies, and (in one large European study) were associated with an increase in aggressive prostate cancer. Natural is better.
- For patients with IBS (primarily diarrhea) and frequent headaches, consider a low-gluten diet. I have the patients limit wheat-based bread, cereal, and pasta. There are many gluten-free products available.
- Aspartame may cause headaches in susceptible patients; aspartame is a commonly used sweetener in products such as diet sodas.
- Caffeine enhances the analgesic effects of aspirin (Excedrin) and of nonsteroidal anti-inflammatory drugs. However, overuse of caffeine may lead to medication-overuse headache. We limit caffeine to 150 or 200 mg/day, at most. The average home-brewed cup of coffee has 120–170 mg. Coffee from Starbucks has more caffeine: 23 mg/oz (approximately). Other specialty coffeehouses also serve coffee with a higher caffeine content. Soft drinks have 50–60 mg/cup, while tea has 0 (if herbal) to 50 mg/cup. Excedrin contains 65 mg of caffeine per tablet.
- Learn about, and recognize, personality disorders. Many medical clinics allow a small number of personality disorders to drain much of the clinic's energy. Get others (psychiatrists, etc.) involved and set limits. It "takes a village" to help a person with pain and a personality disorder.
- For depression to improve, it is important to control pain. Likewise, to help pain, we must treat depression. They tend to "fuel" each other.
- Attention-deficit disorder (ADD) in adults is common (4.7% prevalence). Look for it since ADD decreases quality of life and is relatively easy to treat in adults.
- Watch for soft bipolar signs in headache patients who have anxiety and depression. Bipolar disorder tends to be underdiagnosed, and the clinical stakes for

missing it are enormous. Bipolar disorder, primarily mild and soft (bipolar 2 or 3), is seen in as many as 6–8 % of migraineurs. While some of these patients will do well on an antidepressant, it is almost always necessary to add a mood stabilizer. Soft (milder end of the spectrum) bipolar patients with headache often are placed on antidepressants, with predictably poor results.
- We cannot promise patients that their headaches will improve with psychotherapy (as it often does not), but coping with headaches and the stresses that headaches produce is often improved with therapy. Unfortunately, because of stigma, time, and money, only a small minority of patients will actually go to a therapist. However, those who do go will usually benefit. Biofeedback is underutilized and should be offered more often.

## *Strategies and Procedures*

- It helps to view chronic headache as a continuum or spectrum. The "in-between" headaches may not fall neatly into the current tension or migraine categories. Whether these are severe tension or milder migraines, they often respond to the same medications.
- Kindling of the brain is important in depression, seizures, and headache. It is crucial to treat depression to remission, control seizures, and treat headaches. Possibly, if we treat younger patients with frequent headaches fairly aggressively, we may prevent the progression into chronic daily headache.
- The initial history and physical is the best time to consider a differential list of medications, because at that point we have a good grasp of the patient's comorbidities. If we list in the chart all other treatment possibilities (in case our initial medications do not work), later we, or our partners, do not have to reconstruct the entire history with the patients.
- Keep a drug-medication flow chart, which is easy to do with electronic medical records (EMR). Headache patients are constantly having medications stopped and restarted so that, over 10 years, a patient may have been on 50 different medications at various times. It is impossible to piece through 40 progress notes trying to determine what the next best course of action is. A drug-medication flow chart from the beginning would help immensely. For patients, "chronicpaintracker" is a nice app that is easy to use, tracking meds and triggers, along with pain.
- In treating pain patients, utilizing premade stamps or EMR software can be helpful for documenting that a discussion occurred about side effects, risk/benefits, limits, etc. Opioid stamps for each visit include level of pain and functioning, moods, overuse, and physical exam (pupils/gait/speech).
- When dismissing a patient from your practice (for abusive or drug-seeking behavior, or other reasons), do not abandon the patient. Instead, offer three other physicians' names and phone numbers, suggest that you will transfer records, assist in any way to help obtain another physician, and give the patient 1–3 months to find another provider. It is common for dismissed patients to complain to departments of regulation about "abandonment." Many physicians do not (or

cannot), for various reasons, dismiss patients. These physicians tend to be overrun with abusive personality disorder patients. This leads to legal and regulatory problems, as well as physician burnout. Burnout is a crucial concept, and many strategies need to be used to avoid it. These include in-office: limiting patients, dismissing abusive patients, utilizing staff for paperwork and difficult phone calls, etc. Outside of the office, there are a number of strategies to avoid burnout as well.
- While there is the official definition of pain, we prefer, "Pain is what the patient says it is, and it's as bad as the patient says it is."
- This is an updated version of an article that appeared in *Practical Pain Management,* vol 12, Sept 2012.

## Suggested Reading


1. Banos J, Farre M, Macedo A (2008) Placebo response in the prophylaxis of migraine: a meta-analysis. Eur J Pain 12:68–75
2. Cady R, Dodick D et al (2005) Sinus headache: a neurology, otolaryngology, allergy and primary care consensus. Mayo Clin Proc 80(7):908–916
3. Gardner KL (2006) Genetics of migraine: an update. Headache 46(Suppl 1):S19–S24
4. Headache Classification Subcommittee of the International Headache Society (2003) The international classification of headache disorders, 2nd edn. Blackwell, Oxford
5. Koptchuk J (1998) Powerful placebo: the dark side of the randomized control trial. Lancet 351:1722–1725
6. Lipton RB et al (on behalf of the AMPP Advisory Group) (2007) Migraine prevalence, disease burden, and the need for preventive therapy. Neurology 68:343–349
7. Lipton RB, Varon SF, Grosbert B et al (2011) On-abotulinumtoxin A improves quality of life and reduces impact of chronic migraine. Neurology 77(15):1465–1472
8. Mathew NT, Rapoport A, Saper J, Magnus L et al (2001) Efficacy of gabapentin in migraine prophylaxis. Headache 41(2):119–128
9. MIST Migraine Intervention with Starflex Technology Trial (n.d.) Retrieved from Coverage of American College of Cardiology 55th Annual Scientific Session. www.medscape.com. Accessed 14 Nov 2008
10. Phase III Clinical Trial: Botox for Prevention of Chronic Migraine. Results released. September 2009. www.reutershealth.com. Accessed 14 Nov 2008
11. Raskin N (1988) Headache, 2nd edn. Churchill Livingston, New York, p. 153
12. Robbins L Robbins headache clinic. http://www.headachedrugs.com. Accessed 7 March 2012
13. Robbins L (2000) Management of headaches and headache medications, 2nd edn. Springer, New York
14. Robbins L (2004) Frequent triptan use: observations on safety issues. Headache 44:1–5
15. Robbins L (2008–2009) Headache. www.headachedrugs.com. Accessed 17 Nov 2008
16. Robbins L (2008) The bipolar spectrum in migraine, cluster and chronic tension headache patients. US Neurol Dis 3(2), Feb. 2008
17. Robbins L (2009) Long-acting opioids for refractory chronic migraine. Pract Pain Manag 9(5):74–78
18. Robbins L, Goldfein P (2008) Personality disorders and the bipolar spectrum. Pract Pain Manag 8(3):46–50

19. Robbins L, Maides J (1999) Efficacy of preventive medications for chronic daily headache. Am J Pain Manag 9(4):130–133
20. Silberstein S, Lipton R, Dodick D (2007) Wolff's headache and other head pain, 8th edn. Oxford University Press, New York
21. Webster L, Dove B (2007). Avoiding opioid abuse while managing pain. Sunrise River, Minnesota, p. 676

# Chapter 2
# Refractory (Difficult-to-Treat) Headache

## Difficult-to-Treat Chronic Migraine: Outpatient Medication Approaches

Refractory chronic migraine often is a disabling, debilitating, and challenging illness. Patients who have medication overuse headache or psychological comorbidities require a combination of therapeutic approaches.

Patients with refractory chronic migraine (RCM) experience a great deal of disability and the loss of their quality of life (QOL). Chronic migraine (CM) occurs in approximately 2% of the population, but we do not know the epidemiology or rate of occurrence of RCM.

To provide a framework for other physicians and health care providers, the Refractory Headache Special Interest Section (RHSIS) of the American Headache Society (AHS) was formed in 2001. This committee of headache specialists seeks to define a standard of diagnosis for health practitioners and raise awareness of improved treatments for headache.

The definition of CM is outlined in Table 2.1, and the current proposed criteria for the definition of RCM is a work in progress and is summarized in Table 2.2 [95, 96]. The committee may want to add modifiers related to the degree of refractoriness (mild, moderate, or severe). In some patients, RCM improves or resolves over time, whereas in others it worsens. These differences need to be addressed in the definition [42].

### *Challenges of Refractory Migraine*

RCM presents a number of major challenges, with each challenge necessitating a change in approach [42]. These challenges include:

- What role does disability play, and should disability help to define RCM?
- What constitutes resistance to treatment(s)?



L. Robbins, *Advanced Headache Therapy,* DOI 10.1007/978-3-319-13899-2_2

**Table 2.1** Defining chronic migraine. (Based on Refs. [95, 96])

| | | | |
|---|---|---|---|
| A. | Headache (tension-type and/or migraine) on 15 days per month for at least 3 months | | |
| B. | Occurring in a patient who has had at least five attacks fulfilling criteria for 1.1 migraine without aura | | |
| C. | On 8 days per month for at least 3 months, headache has fulfilled C1 and/or C2 below—that is, has fulfilled criteria for pain and associated symptoms of migraine without aura | | |
| | 1. Has at least two of "a" through "d" | | |
| | | a. | Unilateral location |
| | | b. | Pulsating quality |
| | | c. | Moderate or severe pain intensity |
| | | d. | Aggravation by or causing avoidance of routine physical activity (e.g., walking or climbing stairs) |
| | Has at least one of "e" or "f" | | |
| | | e. | Nausea and/or vomiting |
| | | f. | Photophobia and phonophobia |
| | 2. Treated and relieved by triptan(s) or ergot before the expected development of C1 | | |
| D. | No medication overuse and not attributed to another causative disorder | | |

**Table 2.2** Proposed criteria for definition of refractory migraine and refractory chronic migraine. (Based on Ref. [95])

| Criteria | Definition |
|---|---|
| Primary diagnosis | ICHD-II migraine or chronic migraine |
| Refractory | Headaches cause significant interference with function or quality of life despite modification of triggers, lifestyle factors, and adequate trials of acute and preventive medicines with established efficacy |
| | Failed adequate trails of preventive medicines, alone or in combination, from at least two of four drug classes:<br>Beta-blockers<br>Anticonvulsants<br>Tricyclics<br>Calcium channel blockers |
| | Failed both a triptan and DHE intranasal or injectable formulation<br>Failed either nonsteroidal anti-inflammatory drugs or combination analgesics |
| Adequate trial | Period of time during which an appropriate dose of medicine is administered, typically at least 2 months at optimal or maximum tolerated doses, unless terminated early due to adverse effects |
| Modifiers | With or without medication overuse, as defined by ICHD-2<br>With significant disability, as defined by MIDAS > 11 |

*DHE* dihydroergotamine, *ICHD* international classification of headache disorders, *MIDAS* migraine disability assessment

- There are no accepted, identifiable biological marker(s) for RCM. Therefore, how does one diagnose RCM?
- The degree of disease can change over time, improving or worsening. What role does the varying severity play?

- There are various subsets of RCM—posttraumatic headache, RCM with or without medication overuse headache (MOH), RCM with or without major psychiatric comorbidities, etc. How is the diagnosis and treatment affected by these subsets?
- How does the treatment differ for various ages: adolescent versus young adult versus middle age versus older ages?

## *Pathophysiology*

We are just beginning to look beneath the surface of what causes RCM [28]. Some of the issues include:

- What is the role of genetics in drug resistance and inheritance of chronic headaches?
- What structural changes (in white matter or iron deposition) play a role?
- What role does central sensitization and neuroplasticity play?
- How much involvement is peripheral versus central nervous system (CNS)?
- How does MOH affect the structure and function of the nervous system?
- What is the physiologic impact of psychiatric comorbidities? Do depression and/or anxiety fuel the headaches?

Continuing research is critical to answer these questions.

Several risk factors are posited to drive the development of RCM. These include lifestyle issues such as medication overuse, sleep habits, caffeine overuse, and obesity [45]. While pharmacotherapy may be the cornerstone of treatment, other modalities are no less important. The patient must manage his or her triggers with regard to sleep, food, and caffeine intake. Exercise and weight reduction are encouraged. Stress, another major trigger, may be relieved by practicing biofeedback and/or yoga. Depending on the origin of the pain, physical therapy and massage may help. Problems with the teeth, jaw, eyes, and neck should be addressed.

## *Medication Overuse Headache*

MOH is a critical issue that must be addressed early in the treatment of any form of headache [44]. The overuse of abortive migraine medication, used at the onset of a headache, is a major risk factor for the progression of migraine into RCM. Some patients have medication overuse without an increase in headache. In others, overuse of abortive medications is the principal cause of the headaches.

The criteria for diagnosing MOH are listed in Table 2.3. Note that the headache progresses, instead of subsiding, over time, and the calls for prescription refills will become more frequent with the progression. When treating patients with MOH, the offending drugs will need to be withdrawn or limited. While we do not know, with any certainty, the percentage of RCM patients in whom MOH is a major contributor,

**Table 2.3** Medication overuse headache

| |
|---|
| Headache present on > 15 days/month |
| Regular overuse, > 10 days/month or 15 days/month, depending on the medication type<br>The overuse is for at least 3 months |
| Headache has developed or markedly worsened during medication overuse |

we know that MOH should be one of the first considerations when a patient presents with worsening headaches.

While medication overuse is common, not all overusers suffer from increased headaches as a result of the abortive medications. The current definition of MOH conflates medication overuse with MOH, and, as a result, many patients are incorrectly labeled as having MOH.

## *Treatments for RCM*

There is no algorithm for migraine treatment. The choices of medication will vary for each patient, depending on headache severity and comorbidities. For an RCM patient, the choice of therapy depends on a number of variables, including age, psychiatric comorbidities (for more on psychiatric comorbidities, see related article), tendency towards addiction, sleep, medical conditions, etc. Comorbidities often steer where we go with medications: Conditions such as irritable bowel syndrome (IBS), fatigue, and psychiatric conditions have to be considered. Of course, the familiarity and confidence with a particular therapy on the part of the treating physician plays a major role in selection. It is also crucial to resolve medication overuse, and eliminate rebound in all RCM patients. For the remainder of this chapter, the author has highlighted a number of possible approaches (opioids, onabotulinum toxin, daily or frequent triptans, stimulants, monamine oxidase inhibitors (MAOIs), injections, and miscellaneous), some of which may be combined.

## *Opioids*

In my practice, long-acting opioids (LAOs) are the most commonly used approach for RCM. The best candidate for LAOs is the person who has done well on short-acting opioids (SAOs) and who does not have characteristics of a personality disorder (PD).

### Phases in Opioid Use

There are three distinct phases in the use of opioids. The first phase is the initiation of treatment. This includes the initial screening and risk assessment, the doctor's decision as to which opioid to use, and the doctor–patient discussion and signing of an opioid agreement. Prior to initiation of LAOs, an assessment of the following should be done: pain level, moods, social and family functioning, work status, physical functioning, and activities of daily living [27].

The intermediate phase comprises the diligent monitoring of the patient while he/she is on the opioid. This must include ongoing assessment of the patient's pain level and overall functioning, with a watchful eye for signs of abuse. On return visits, the physical exam needs to assess for slurring of words, abnormal gait, and pupillary abnormalities. Do not assume that low-risk patients will never abuse the opioids. During the maintenance phase of opioid prescribing, it is remarkable how many seemingly low-risk patients misuse the drugs.

Patients usually respond fairly quickly to an opioid; if they have not responded by 2–4 weeks on a low dose, there usually will not be an adequate response [88]. If patients do not report an improvement in functioning, or if functioning declines, consideration should be given to withdrawal the opioid. Some patients have an improvement in pain but a decline in physical activity, possibly due to sedation or other opioid-related side effects.

The third phase is switching or withdrawing the opioids when abuse has occurred or there is lack of efficacy. Withdrawing or switching an opioid may be exceedingly difficult in some patients. Each of these phases involves a learning curve on the part of the practitioner and proper documentation by staff members.

In my experience, using higher doses of the opioid rarely works out in the long term. Higher doses place the patient at an increased risk for addiction and abuse as well as complications from withdrawal. It may be thought that, given the great variation in individual responses, the opioid should be increased or "pushed" to whatever level is beneficial. However, medical and regulatory considerations should be limiting factors in keeping the opioid dose at a low level.

The choice of opioid may be key; some have been shown to have less abuse potential. The once- or twice-daily, long-acting morphine preparations have not been subjected to widespread abuse. Methadone may be more effective than some of the other medications, but has a litany of problems associated with it. Besides the social stigma, high protein binding is a risk, which may lead to irregular drug levels, difficulty with withdrawal, and an increased risk for sudden death [64]. If methadone is used, it should be started at a very low dose of no more than 5–10 mg a day, and titrated slowly. Patients placed on methadone require close monitoring, and other sedatives must be reduced or discontinued. The usual dosing range in my practice is:

- Methadone, 5–40 mg per day
- Morphine, 20–90 mg per day
- Oxycodone, 20–60 mg per day
- Hydrocodone, 15–40 mg per day

Some type of written opioid agreement should be part of the doctor–patient alliance, although there is a lack of evidence that these agreements do much good for the majority of the patients. There is no standard opioid contract; practices should adapt one for their own purposes. There are several resources on opioid agreements (www.painmed.org; www.ampainsoc.org; www.fsmb.org; www.usdoj.gov/dea). In addition, there is an excellent article on agreement contracts by Fishman [25].

The treatment of breakthrough pain is controversial. Most of the breakthrough studies have been concerned with cancer pain, where the average number of breakthroughs is 4 per 24 h [111]. For patients with noncancer breakthrough pain, such as chronic daily headache, I tend to minimize the total opioid and avoid layering pain medicines on top of each other. Prescribing short-acting medications for chronic headaches greatly increases the abuse rate. The occasional patient can remain on a low dose of the LAO, with one or two SAOs per day, but, in general, clinicians should try to avoid SAOs.

## Long-Acting Opioids

The following summarizes certain LAO studies and describes guidelines for using LAOs in chronic migraineurs.

In 1997, Saper and associates assessed refractory chronic daily headache with scheduled LAOs, particularly methadone [91]. There was a small subset of patients who did well. Subsequently, Saper and his associates soured on the use of the opioids.

Similar results were obtained from Rothrock [87]. An unpublished study from Rothrock indicated that of the CM patients who were responsive at 2 months to methadone treatment, more than 70 % continued to maintain a response at 1 year [88]. Rothrock found that patients tend to either respond to relatively low doses or not at all. His studies also indicated that virtually all of the positive responders, when tapered off of the methadone, relapsed into their frequent headache patterns [88].

In 2007, our group evaluated 115 patients with RCM who were treated with LAOs during a 6-year period. This was a select group of patients who previously had all done well on SAOs. Avoidance of opioid-induced hyperalgesia (OIH) is important in patients taking opioids in the long term; however, all of the patients in this study already had been on SAOs for at least 1 year [76].

Sixty-five percent of the patients did well for at least 9 months on the opioid. This was a significantly higher rate of success than that found in a previous study (13 %) that used a different standard of success [65]. The average duration of use of the opioid was 4.5 years. Forty-four percent of the patients reported adverse events. Patients with an increased chance of success included younger patients, patients with high coping skills, and those without a history of opioid abuse. Predictors of failure were comorbid PDs, older age, and, in particular, previous abuse of the SAOs. In this study, anxiety, depression, bipolar depression, attention deficit disorder (ADD), exercise, work status, disability, fatigue, and cigarette smoking did not significantly change the long-term outcome.

## SAOs Versus LAOs

The term SAO generally refers not only to how long a drug carries the desired effect but also the speed of onset of the drug and how fast it drops off toward the end of the dose. Quick onsets and fast drop-offs are major determinants for abuse [36].

**Table 2.4** The pros and cons of long-acting opioids

| *The advantages of long-acting opioids include* |
|---|
| Avoidance of the "end-of-the-dose" phenomenon, with mini-withdrawals throughout the day |
| Consistent dosing one or two times daily, which decreases the obsession with the next dose |
| Maintenance of stable blood levels |
| Avoidance of acetaminophen, aspirin, and NSAIDs that are included in many short-acting preparations |
| Probable diminished risk of significant abuse |
| Better compliance, with less psychological dependency on the drug |
| *The disadvantages of long-acting opioids include* |
| Social stigma |
| Fatigue and constipation |
| Difficulty in obtaining scripts, with no refills available |
| Need for frequent office visits and monitoring |
| Risk of opioid-induced hyperalgesia |
| Risk of abuse, although probably less than with short-acting opioids |
| Interactions with other sedating drugs and alcohol |
| Risk for overdose |

*NSAID* nonsteroidal anti-inflammatory drug

SAOs are not necessarily quick-onset medications. Most oral SAO tablets are slow to take effect. A short duration of action then leads to frequent administration by the patient, and overuse may occur. However, it has not been proven conclusively that SAOs lead to more abuse than LAOs. Although certain long-acting drugs have been easily abused, such as oxycodone CR, it is the person, not the drug, who governs abuse. While some abusers have only one drug of choice, many will tend to abuse a succession of drugs.

Several previous studies have evaluated daily opioids for severe chronic daily headache [63, 87, 91]. While success rates have been relatively low, they represent patients who have failed the usual ministrations, and who have few options available. Table 2.4 outlines the advantages and disadvantages of LAOs.

## Opioid Abuse

Opioid abuse is much more common than true addiction. In general, using opioids for therapeutic reasons other than pain constitutes abuse. In a headache practice, the most common reasons for abuse are using the opioids to alleviate moods, anxiety, or depression.

Patients in our previous study were assessed for behaviors typical of opioid abuse or overuse. The criteria that we used included: early refill requests, dose escalations, insistence on increasing doses, abusive treatment of the staff regarding refills, false reports of stolen or lost medications, using the opioid for depression or anxiety, using the opioid for other pains not discussed with the physician, receiving similar medication from other physicians, unexpected or abnormal urine screening test results, using illicit drugs or alcohol, missing, canceling, or refusing appointments, selling the drugs, obtaining opioids from nonmedical arenas, frequent emergency room (ER) visits for opioids, hoarding, forging or altering scripts, borrowing or stealing similar medications from family and friends, physical signs of overuse or addiction, and calls to the physician from family members with concerns about patient overuse [11, 110].

There is a range of abuse, from the person who samples his spouse's codeine prescription once in a while to the addict who obtains hundreds of opioid tablets from the Internet. We cannot paint all abusers with one broad brush. Some situations need watching, such as the patient who took her mom's pills because she had excess pain; this behavior is a red flag and the patient may be an abuser. For a different patient, one who already has been prescribed low-dose, long-acting morphine, the discovery of undisclosed opioid prescriptions from other sources must be regarded as severe abuse. In this situation, discontinuation of the opioids is necessary.

It is not always clear how serious the abuse is. Minor aberrant behaviors often are overlooked. It is not as if any one aberrant behavior warrants immediate discontinuation of an opioid, but most of the serious overuse situations follow a number of previous minor abuse occurrences. Physicians must pay attention to red flags, particularly those that arise early in the relationship with the patient. In my experience, pain patients who raise objections to urine tests usually have a drug problem. Specimen collections should be random and not scheduled. Urine testing serves two purposes: To identify other substances that are present but should not be and to measure the levels of the prescribed substance for compliance. When there is no opioid present, there sometimes is laboratory error or test insensitivity, but it may be that the patient has been binging early on and has run out of drugs before the visit [30]. Another possibility is that the patient is selling the drugs.

In those who self-medicate, a drug is used for a purpose other than the intended one, such as using an opioid as a mood stabilizer or enhancer. Opioids can be both calming and stimulating, often giving a brief burst of energy followed by a tranquil period. Chemical coping is all too common, but is poorly understood and under-researched [62]. All addicts are chemical copers to some degree, but not all people who cope chemically are addicts. The person who uses one or two pills of hydrocodone a day for stress and anxiety is not an addict by definition but is certainly using chemicals to cope. The severe patients basically live for the drug; their lives are controlled by its procurement, and they have few coping skills outside of using the drug [56]. They will self-escalate their drug use, particularly during periods of high stress.

As much as 35 % of patients with chronic pain may fall under the definition of chemical copers [37]. There are gender differences, with women using the substances primarily for anxiety, stress, and depression. Women are at somewhat of an increased risk for chemically coping than are men [56]. Men may use the drugs for anxiety and depression, but they also use them out of boredom, particularly when they are disabled by their pain. For some men, there is a strong relationship between substance abuse and sensation seeking [56].

While physical dependence and tolerance are to be expected with long-term opioid use, addiction is not. Addiction constitutes a biologic and behavioral disease. Most abusers can stop using the drug when harm occurs, but an addict cannot. Whether a patient with previous addictions should be treated with LAOs is a complicated issue. It should be approached on a case-by-case basis and depends on a number of factors. Among the considerations:

- What substances were abused?
- How many years has the patient been clean?
- Has the patient successfully completed treatment for addiction?
- What is the quality of the patient's support system?
- Does the patient have any comorbid psychiatric conditions [110]?
- What are the patient's risk factors?

Previous studies have indicated that risk factors for opioid abuse include cigarette smoking, previous drug abuse, a strong family history of drug abuse, stress, young age, early sexual abuse, poor support, low level of functioning due to headache or other pain, pain embellishment, and certain psychiatric conditions [6, 22, 94].

A National Institute of Mental Health (NIMH) analysis identified certain problems that carried an increased risk for substance abuse [54]. Of patients with anxiety, 25 % had a substance use problem, as did 33 % of those with obsessive–compulsive disorder (OCD), and 61 % in the bipolar I category. Unipolar depression also carried a higher risk, but not as much as bipolar disorder. Among PD patients, Webster found that 84 % of those with antisocial PDs were substance abusers [110]. Also, patients with somatization are probably at a higher risk. In a study by Biederman et al., untreated attention-deficit hyperactivity disorder (ADHD) in older adolescent boys carried a 75 % risk for substance abuse, whereas those with treated ADHD in this age group had a 25 % risk. The boys without ADHD had an 18 % overall abuse rate [7].

As noted, our study indicated that those with PDs were at an increased risk for abuse but that other psychiatric conditions did not lead to more abuse [76].

## Successful Management of LAOs

The physician must have knowledge and experience in the use of these drugs. The patient has to be reliable and well-known to the practitioner. Many of the problems occur with new patients; it is prudent to wait several visits before prescribing LAOs—after the physician can establish that there has been little or no previous abuse.

In our practice, patients must have demonstrated an adequate response to SAOs. To avoid OIH, we restrict use to patients who have received SAOs for 1 year or more. The patient must truly be refractory to the typical ministrations, with multiple adequate trials of the usual preventive medications. Previous abuse of opioids should exclude patients from this treatment approach. In this author's view, previous abuse of SAOs almost always leads to abuse of the LAOs. Pseudoaddiction certainly is encountered, but it seems to be rare in headache patients. Be wary of the patient who claims he or she can tolerate almost no medications except for opioids.

In older patients, particularly those over age 65, the brain has lost the ability to do the "neuronal gymnastics" necessary for the development of tolerance to the analgesic effect. Therefore, older patients may remain on the same low dose for a number of years. In contrast, the use of opioids in patients under 30 years of age should be restricted because younger patients are more likely to develop tolerance to the analgesic effects. If a younger patient fulfills all the requirements, such as truly being refractory, is normal psychologically, and is at low risk for addiction, he or she may be the exception to the age rule.

Management of those with CM involves a biopsychosocial approach. Patients must not rely on the drug to function. While medications may be a mainstay of therapy, other interventions must be employed. Active coping should be strongly encouraged with each visit, and may involve a variety of approaches, including seeing a psychotherapist, physical therapist, or other practitioners, or using self-help approaches such as exercise or biofeedback. Passive coping is a major predictor of disability in chronic pain patients. Patients who rely only on opioids have less of a chance of sustaining long-term relief. Even though pharmacotherapy is the cornerstone of treatment, it is only part of a more comprehensive plan.

## *Botulinum Toxin Injections*

Onabotulinum toxin type A (Botox, Xeomin, and Dysport) has been used as a migraine and chronic daily headache preventive since the 1990s [5]. Botox is the only brand that is Food and Drug Administration (FDA) indicated for CM.

The results of studies have varied widely. Two phase III studies (Phase III Research Evaluating Migraine Prophylaxis Therapy (PREEMPT) 1 and 2) with 1384 CM patients found onabotulinum toxin (specifically the brand Botox) useful for improving functioning and reducing disability. One of the studies was very positive in reducing headache days [58]. The preponderance of evidence points to onabotulinum toxin as being safe and efficacious, and this author concurs.

There are a number of possible explanations as to why onabotulinum toxin may alleviate pain. One of its mechanisms of action is that it is anti-inflammatory at the neuronal level. Onabotulinum toxin may block the release of substance P. More importantly, it may also inhibit the level of secretion of calcitonin gene-related peptide (CGRP) [5]. CGRP has been recognized as a key inflammatory mediator, a vital cog in the cascade leading to headache. Efforts are underway to develop drugs that are CGRP antagonists. Onabotulinum toxin also may block the release of certain other neuropeptides that contribute to the "inflammatory soup." This neuropeptide blockage and onabotulinum toxin's inhibitory effects on the excitatory neurotransmitter glutamate result in a lessening of peripheral sensitization.

With the use of onabotulinum toxin, there is also a decrease in central sensitization [55]. Relatively few other compounds have an effect on central sensitization, which is so vital to the pathophysiology of CM.

As with a number of migraine treatments, the results of onabotulinum toxin studies vary. A number of variables may explain some of the differences, including [5]:

- Headache severity, chronicity, and degree of refractoriness
- Medication overuse
- Different types of pain ("imploding" vs. "exploding")
- Different methods of assessing outcomes

Different numbers of units of onabotulinum toxin used and different locations of injections.

In a number of onabotulinum toxin studies, the high placebo response rate has been difficult to overcome in proving efficacy. The optimal mechanics of onabotulinum toxin administration are still a work in progress [14, 97]. The FDA's indicated dose for Botox is 155 units, administered in 31 injections about the head. Some patients do well with much less, which is off-label.

For some patients, we "chase the pain" and administer additional injections around the area of pain, which is also off-label. For those with occipital pain, posterior injections may be very helpful. If patients do not respond to the first treatment, it is worthwhile to repeat onabotulinum toxin at least once more. Onabotulinum toxin is expensive but relatively safe. It may be combined with various medication approaches.

Side effects to onabotulinum toxin tend to be minimal; occasionally patients experience a mild droop of one eye. Some have reported numbness or other sensations around the areas of injection. Generalized weakness should not occur with the low doses that are used. On occasion, patients experience an increase in headaches for a short time.

## *Daily or Frequent Triptans*

It has been over 20 years since triptans were first introduced, and they appear to be much safer than was originally thought. Very few serious adverse events have been reported, considering that more than 100 million patients have taken triptans. Several studies have described the use of daily triptans for the preventive treatment of chronic daily headache [76, 73]. Some patients respond only to triptan medications—sumatriptan (Imitrex, Alsuma, others), naratriptan (Amerge, others), rizatriptan (Maxalt, others), almotriptan (Axert), zolmitriptan (Zomig, others), frovatriptan (Frova), and eletriptan (Relpax). Zecuity is a sumatriptan skin patch.

Short-lasting adverse events are often encountered with triptan use. These include paresthesias, fatigue, chest heaviness, and jaw or neck discomfort [15]. Chest symptoms are, with rare exceptions, not of cardiovascular origin. Echocardiography and electrocardiography generally have been normal after triptan use, even in the presence of chest symptoms.

The primary issue with frequent triptan use, assuming rebound headache is not present, is long-term adverse events. Chronic ischemic changes, valvular abnormalities, and fibrosis are theoretical considerations. Cardiac ischemia due to triptan use is rare [15], and, despite widespread triptan use, the number of adverse cardiac events has been limited. These risks have not been systematically studied, however. The number of patients throughout the world who have used triptans on a near-daily basis is unknown. Until these patients have been studied, it is reasonable and prudent to do cardiac monitoring, as well as hematologic tests.

To study the cardiac safety of frequent triptan use, we studied patient who "on their own" had discovered that daily use of a triptan would alleviate headaches for most or all of the day [73]. Most patients in the study had a long history of headaches that were refractory to usual medications. Most of the patients had been using frequent triptans, prescribed by their primary care physician. A minority of our patients had increased the amount of triptans they used on their own.

Patients were withdrawn from triptans to determine if rebound headache was present. The only patients who continued on triptans were those who had been determined truly to be refractory to other approaches, experienced no or minimal side effects, had rebound headaches excluded, and signed a "Frequent Triptan Informed Consent" form. A summary of patient dose and usage can be found in Table 2.5.

Routine laboratory (hematologic) tests, including complete blood counts and chemistries, were done, and no abnormalities were felt to be due to triptans. Electrocardiograms (ECGs) were performed on all of the 118 patients, and 8 patients (7 %) had abnormal findings that were determined not to be from the triptan. Echocardiograms (with Doppler) were done on 57 of the 118 patients (48 %), and 10 of those patients (17 %) had abnormal findings. The attending cardiologist did not feel that any of these abnormalities were due to triptan use. Twenty patients underwent stress tests, and all were normal [73].

Of the 118 patients, 9 felt that the triptans contributed to fatigue; 5 had mild chest tightness at times that was possibly due to the triptans, but cardiac disease was ruled out; and 3 felt that the triptans contributed to nausea [73].

Because the patients in the study decided to use triptans on a daily basis on their own, adverse events would be expected to be low. If patients were not tolerating the medication well or were having significant adverse effects, they would not choose to continue the triptan on a frequent basis. There were no adverse consequences from frequent triptan use over a prolonged period. So, frequent triptan use is not ideal, but may actually be safer than some other approaches. Of course, patients must accept the possibility of the (rare) serious side effect.

## *Stimulants*

When prescribed for headache patients, stimulants may be beneficial for various comorbidities, such as ADHD, depression, and fatigue. In addition, stimulants do not cause the weight gain that is seen with a number of other headache preventive

**Table 2.5** Characteristics of daily triptan use among 118 patients

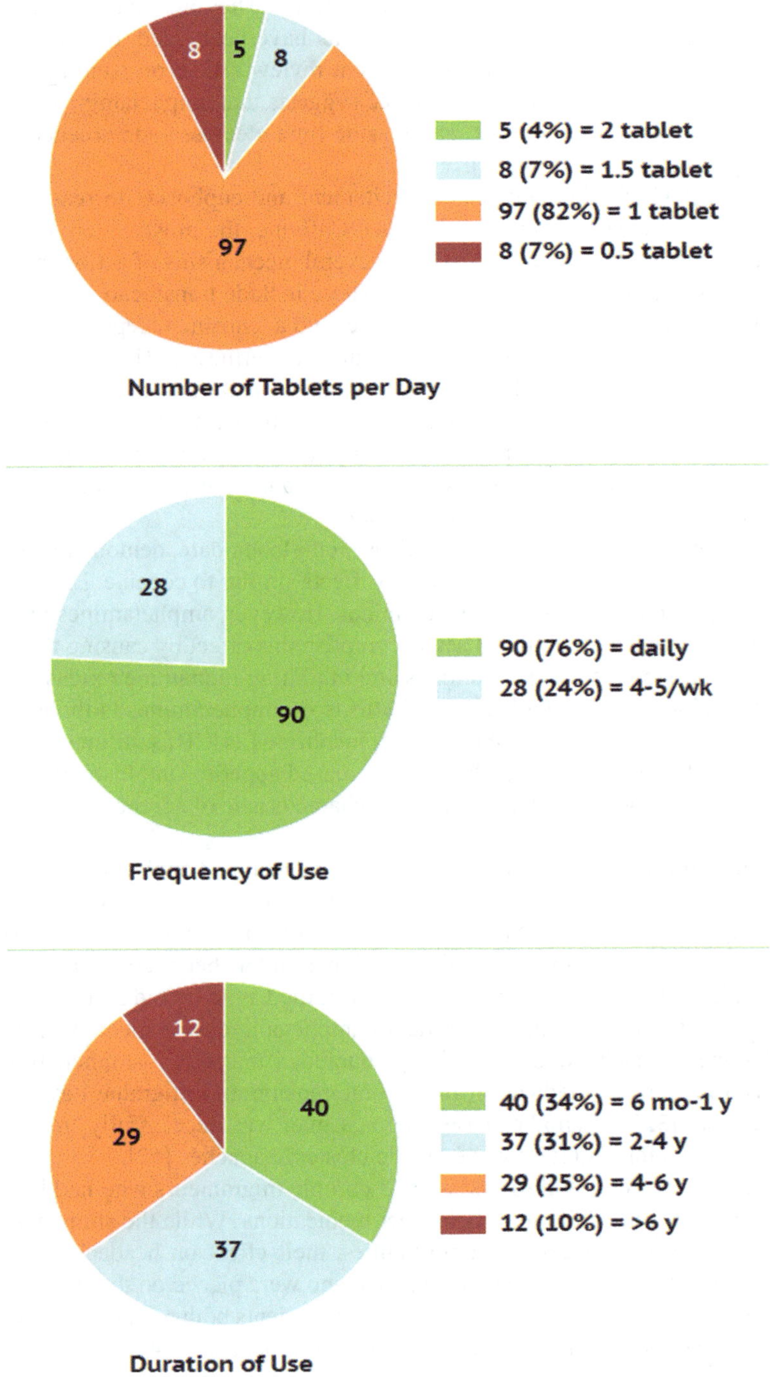

medications. Amphetamines have been shown to possess intrinsic analgesic properties, primarily through brain catecholamine activity. They also intensify the analgesic effects of certain opioids [21]. Stimulants have been used to counteract the sedation encountered by opioids. An excellent review article on stimulants as adjuncts for opioids concluded that "evidence suggests that amphetamine drugs may enhance the effect of opioids and, at the same time, decrease somnolence and increase cognitive performance [17]."

As a group, CNS stimulants cause excitement and euphoria, decrease feelings of fatigue, and increase motor activity [24]. Caffeine, the most widely consumed stimulant in the world, is believed to have several mechanisms of action in the prefrontal cortex and other areas of the brain. These include translocation of extracellular calcium, inhibition of phosphodiesterase, and adenosine receptor antagonism, resulting in decreased fatigue and increased mental alertness [24].

Nicotine, the active ingredient in tobacco, specifically stimulates nicotinic receptors in the autonomic ganglia, resulting in euphoria, arousal, relaxation, and improved attention, learning, problem solving, and reaction time [24]. However, in very high doses, nicotine causes blockade of autonomic ganglia, resulting in respiratory depression and severe hypotension.

Amphetamine and its derivatives, such as methylphenidate, demonstrate indirect CNS and peripheral nervous system (PNS) effects similar to cocaine. Like cocaine, they initially increase levels of catecholamines. However, amphetamines do this by a different mechanism of action. They accomplish this effect by causing the release of intracellular stores of catecholamines and inhibiting monamine oxidase (MAO) [24]. The major cause of the behavioral effects of amphetamines is thought to be due more to release of dopamine than norepinephrine [24]. This, ultimately, results in increased alertness, decreased fatigue, decreased appetite, and insomnia, as well as the usual "fight or flight" response that is characteristic of adrenergic stimulation in the PNS.

Amphetamines have been known to possess independent analgesic activity, possibly due to release of norepinephrine. The effect was felt to be about the same as that of ibuprofen. As noted, stimulants may potentiate the analgesic actions of opioids [17]. The most commonly studied combination has been dextroamphetamine and morphine. Methylphenidate also has been studied as an opioid adjunctive medication. In one small study, the use of dextroamphetamine for patients with tension and migraine headache was assessed. It concluded that dextroamphetamine was viable as a preventive medication for chronic tension and migraine headaches in some subjects [32]. In another case report, a man was successfully treated with methylphenidate for his refractory episodic cluster headaches [52].

One of our previous studies assessed 73 chronic migraineurs who had been prescribed stimulants in addition to their other medications. While the stimulants were primarily prescribed for certain comorbidities, their effect on headaches was also assessed. Seventy-five percent of the patients who were placed on the stimulants remained on them for at least 9 months; 34 % of the patients both remained on the stimulants and reported positive efficacy with regard to headache; 41 % of the patients suffered at least 1 adverse event, whereas only 2 patients abused the stimulant [86].

Advantages of stimulants include enhanced cognition and alertness, with no weight gain. Disadvantages primarily revolve around the side effects, such as anxiety or insomnia. Abuse certainly may occur, but it is uncommon in adults. Stimulants should be considered in patients with certain comorbidities. The few studies conducted to date have indicated a positive role for stimulants, but further studies on stimulants for headache would help to clarify that role.

## *Monoamine Oxidase Inhibitors*

For those with RCM and unipolar depression, monoamine oxidase inhibitors (MAOIs) may be of help. MAOIs sometimes are effective for treatment-resistant depression [40]. They are also effective for alleviating anxiety. MAOIs were commonly prescribed in the 1980s, but with the advent of selective serotonin reuptake inhibitors (SSRIs) and triptans, they fell out of favor. The available literature on MAOIs for headache treatment dates to the 1970s and 1980s. For a select group of RCM patients, the MAOIs greatly enhance QOL. At this point, I believe that MAOIs are underused.

The traditional, classical MAOIs form an irreversible complex with the enzyme monoamine oxidase. Monoamine oxidase is located in a number of tissues, including the brain. The mechanism of action is most likely receptor-mediated pre- and postsynaptic events, not simply an increase in serotonin [40]. The traditional MAOI phenelzine has been the one most commonly used for headache.

The transdermal selegiline patch (Emsam) is a selective MAO-B inhibitor that does not require patients to eat a tyramine-restricted diet, at least in the lowest (6-mg) dose. Another nontraditional reversible MAOI is moclobemide, which is not available in the USA. Moclobemide has fewer dietary and medication restrictions than the classic MAOIs. The efficacy of these nontraditional MAOIs is not as clearly established as the more traditional MAOIs (phenelzine) [41].

Careful patient selection is crucial when using the MAOIs. Patients need to carefully observe the restrictions on diet and medications. I usually prescribe low doses of phenelzine and start patients with 15 mg at night, increasing after 1 week to 30 mg at night. If no response is noted after 3–4 weeks, I usually increase the dose to 45 mg at night; 75 mg is the usual maximum dose. By always taking the MAOI at night, the patient is less likely to encounter a food interaction. Side effects include insomnia, weight gain, sedation, and orthostatic hypotension. The MAOIs have a reputation as being somewhat dangerous and difficult to use, but they usually are well tolerated.

The previous MAOI diets were overly restrictive. The risk of most foods was based on anecdotal cases. Newer evidence-based diets are easier to follow (Table 2.6) [60]. The hypertensive crisis that may occur with a food interaction is due to a number of factors, primarily the amount of tyramine absorbed into the bloodstream. The tyramine content of food has been difficult to accurately establish. When patients consume phenelzine at night in low doses and avoid the major tyramine-rich foods, interactions are less likely.

**Table 2.6** Sunnybrook health center MAOI diet

| Food group | Food to avoid | Food allowed |
|---|---|---|
| *Cheese* | Mature or aged cheese, casseroles made with these cheeses; all others except listed in “allowed” column | Fresh cottage, cream, and ricotta cheese and processed cheese slices; all fresh milk products |
| *Meat, fish, poultry* | Fermented/dry sausage, pepperoni, salami, mortadella, improperly stored meat, fish, and poultry | All fresh packaged or processed meat, fish, and poultry, stored in refrigerator and eaten as soon as possible |
| *Fruits and vegetables* | Fava or broad bean pods, banana peel | Banana pulp, all others, except those listed in “avoid” column |
| *Alcoholic beverages* | All tap beer | Alcohol: no more than two domestic or canned beers or four oz. wine a day |
| *Miscellaneous foods* | Marmite yeast concentrate, sauerkraut, soy sauce, and soy condiments | Other yeast extracts, soy milk |

*MAOI* monoamine oxidase inhibitor

Serotonin syndrome may occur due to the administration of serotonergic drugs (i.e., SSRIs) and MAOIs. Other drugs that should be avoided include amphetamines, sympathomimetics, pseudoephedrine, certain opioids (meperidine), dextromethorphan, and others. Most triptans are not combined with MAOIs, but low doses of triptans (frovatriptan and several others) may be used with caution.

For patients suffering from both refractory chronic headache and treatment-resistant depression, MAOIs may offer some measure of hope and are not as dangerous as their reputation might imply.

## Injections and Nerve Blocks

Various injections and blocks are used for refractory headache. For frontal headaches, sphenopalatine ganglion (SPG) blocks may be useful. Posteriorly, occipital injections are used. For cervical and occipital pain, various cervical blocks or injections may be helpful.

### SPG Blocks

For frontal headache, blocking the SPG can be helpful. This has been done for 100 years, but three newer devices make it easy to do. These are the SphenoCath, the Tx360, and the Allevio SPG device. Each of these shrinks the time required from 1 h to a few minutes. SPG blocks, usually performed with bupivacaine, are safe, with few reported adverse events. For (frontal) CMs, the blocks are helpful if done 2 (or 3) days per week for several weeks.

### Cervical Blocks/Injections

Various cervical procedures may be helpful, particularly if cervicogenic headache is present. When the pain is primarily in the posterior occipital area, and/or the neck, these procedures may be beneficial. Cervical epidurals may provide temporary relief. Facet injections often are useful as well. If the temporary blocks help, then procedures that are longer lasting might be more beneficial.

### Occipital Nerve Blocks

For posterior head pain, blocking one or both occipital nerves may help, at least for a period of time. Occipital blocks are the treatment of choice when occipital neuralgia is present. If the pain is anterior and posterior, combining SPG and occipital blocks may provide relief.

## *Polypharmacy*

Rational polypharmacy is commonly used for RCM. Comorbidities influence medications selection. Two (or more) preventives may be more effective than one. However, we also strive to minimize the number of medications used. If a patient is hypertensive and depressed, an angiotensin-receptor blocker plus an antidepressant might lessen the headache. Weight gain often is a concern, and with these patients, we avoid certain medications (valproate, amitriptyline, propranolol, etc.). Many RCM patients complain of being chronically tired. A number of headache medications may exacerbate fatigue. For patients with IBS, we would attempt to choose medications that may help treat the IBS and the headache. Some medications may help the diarrhea of IBS, but constipation tends to be a difficult problem in patients with IBS and headache because a number of headache drugs exacerbate constipation. Unfortunately, there are no algorithms that apply to complicated RCM patients. Each patient, with their comorbidities, is unique.

## *Miscellaneous*

Methylergonovine (Methergine) is a smooth muscle constrictor that primarily is used to stop bleeding after childbirth. Methylergonovine is useful for a small number of RCM patients. The usual dose is one tablet three times daily. Triptans usually are not used concurrently. Availability has been a problem.

Muscle relaxants occasionally help those with RCM. We usually stick with non-addicting muscle relaxants, such as baclofen (Lioresal) or cyclobenzaprine (Flexeril, Amrix). Fatigue is a common side effect. Another muscle relaxant, metaxalone (Skelaxin), minimizes fatigue. These agents may be beneficial for treating insomnia as well. Many patients use low doses of these (half a tablet at a time).

Memantine (Namenda) is a drug used for the treatment of Alzheimer's disease and dementia. Memantine is an *N*-methyl-D-aspartate receptor antagonist that may be helpful for pain management. Memantine is a safe, well-tolerated drug. The usual dose of memantine is 14–21 mg per day.

## *New Developments*

New approaches, such as transcranial magnetic stimulation (TMS), are becoming available. In December 2013, the US FDA approved the first TMS device specifically for the management of migraine (Cerena, eNeura TMS). According to the FDA, nearly 38% of subjects who used the Cerena (eNeura) TMS when they had migraine pain were pain-free 2 h after using the device compared to about 17% of patients in the control group. After 24 h, nearly 34% of the Cerena (eNeura) TMS users were pain-free compared to 10% in the control group [26]. TMS has few side effects and has been in testing for 10 years. Patients can have a unit at home that delivers several quick, magnetic pulses to the occipital cortex in the brain. Over time, we will see how effective TMS is for severe headaches. Studies are very promising.

Occipital nerve stimulation has been beneficial for a small number of RCM patients. Techniques of implantation have improved, but the technical challenges need to be overcome. The leads tend to migrate away from the occipital nerve, for example. While it is invasive, expensive, and associated with frequent side effects, nerve stimulation is viable for a small number of patients. Other nerves (such as the supraorbital) have also been the target of nerve stimulation.

In pharmacotherapy, there are a number of emerging compounds that may eventually come to market. These include newer preventive techniques, such as a monthly injection of a CGRP antibody. CGRP preventives are very promising.

## *Conclusion*

RCM often is a disabling and debilitating illness. We face major challenges in attempting to define RCM. The definition must allow for severity of illness; also, degrees of refractoriness may change over time.

Other major areas of study within RCM include pathophysiologic mechanisms, the role of medication overuse, a search for biomarkers, psychological comorbidities, nonmedication approaches, and pharmacotherapy.

Patients with RCM who have MOH or psychological comorbidities require a combination of approaches. It "takes a village" to help those with severe, refractory headaches, and we need to guide the patient into comprehensive treatments. There are a number of viable therapeutic approaches, a number of approaches are presented in this chapter. However, we desperately need breakthrough medications and technologies that can prevent headache pain. Note this is an updated version of an article that appeared in the September 2014 issue of *Practical Pain Management*.

## RCM: The Use of LAOs

Study results for a group of difficult-to-treat migraineurs provide a basis for determining efficacy and guidelines for the use of long-term opioids in this population.

Many patients with CM are refractory to our usual therapies [83]. Medication choices for the refractory chronic migraineur are limited and include polypharmacy with several preventives, MAOIs, botulinum toxin type A (Botox) and opioids, among others [67]. Each of these pharmacologic approaches helps a limited number of patients.

There have been a number of studies on LAOs as a treatment for refractory chronic daily headache [63, 87, 91]. Earlier studies focused on the use of low doses of methadone and a small minority of patients who did well in the long term. Several studies reported better success rates with other opioids, such as oxycodone CR or long-acting morphine preparations [66]. This suggested that, for the difficult-to-treat patient, this approach may be worthwhile, despite the difficulties in prescribing daily opioids.

The current study evaluated LAOs for those who had done well with SAOs for an extended period. These patients had been prescribed SAOs for significant periods in the past. Certain comorbidities were evaluated to assess if they could have predictive value as to who would do well with the opioid and who would fail. These comorbidities were also used to assess risk for abuse.

### *Study Design*

This retrospective study was conducted at a single US headache clinic. Data were collected via chart review, patient diary, and patient interview. Patients who had been prescribed LAOs during the 6-year period 2002–2007 were assessed.

Patients kept a headache diary and used a ten-point visual analog scale to measure severity. Functional status was assessed with each visit. If adequate functioning was not maintained, the patient was usually withdrawn from the opioid. During each visit, the following were assessed in addition to functioning:

Pain level
Brief physical exam
Side effects of the opioid
Overuse/abuse behaviors

### *Patient Characteristics*

For the study 115 patients were evaluated (87 female, 28 male, age range 23–77). All patients had been diagnosed as having RCM [96]. They had longstanding daily headaches that caused significant functional impairment or decreased QOL. Each patient had failed multiple trials of preventive medicines. In addition, they had little or no relief from abortive medications (triptans, nonsteroidal anti-inflammatory drugs (NSAIDs), dihydroergotamine (DHE), etc.) While attempts were made to minimize MOH, patients with this condition were not excluded from using the LAOs. Virtually every one of these patients would qualify as RCM utilizing the 2008 proposed criteria for definition of refractory migraine and RCM [96].

## *Inclusion Criteria*

Long-time patients at the treating headache clinic with a diagnosis of RCM were included. CM was defined according to the International Headache Society (HIS) criteria [100]. All patients had been prescribed LAOs, including methadone, long-acting forms of morphine or oxycodone, or the fentanyl patch during the years 2002–2007. All patients had previously shown improved functioning and QOL on SAOs. The minimum period of use of the SAOs was 1 year. Thirty-two (28%) of the patients had abused the SAOs to some degree.

## *Primary Outcome Measure: Efficacy*

The primary outcome measure was efficacy of the opioid. Efficacy was determined to be positive (+) if the patient continued on the LAO for at least 9 months and the patient consistently reported a 30% or greater improvement in headache frequency and/or severity over baseline. The baseline of comparison was the 3-month period prior to initiation of the LAO.

## *Secondary Outcome Measures: Definitions and Criteria*

### Opioid Abuse

The term "opioid abuse" is not well-defined in the literature and is rather imprecise. However, we use this term for the study because it encompasses not only true addiction but lesser forms of overuse as well—such as chemical coping [56]. In our current study, patients were labeled as abusers if certain behaviors were severe, persistent, or pervasive. Some of the criteria were felt to be more significant than others. The criteria that we used included: early refill requests; dose escalations; insistence on increasing doses; abusive treatment of the staff regarding refills; false reports of stolen or lost medications; utilizing the opioid for depression or anxiety; using the opioid for other pains not discussed with the physician; receiving similar medication from other physicians; unexpected or abnormal urine screening test results; using illicit drugs or alcohol; repeatedly missing, canceling, or refusing appointments; selling the drugs; obtaining opioids from nonmedical arenas; frequent ER visits for opioids; hoarding, forging, or altering scripts; borrowing or stealing similar medications from family and friends; physical signs of overuse or addiction; and calls to the physician from family members with concerns about patient overuse [141, 110].

### Anxiety

Patients with anxiety disorders included those with generalized anxiety disorder, panic disorder, and OCD. Anxiety was assessed via patient interviews, histories, and the initial anxiety and psychiatric assessment forms. *Diagnostic and Statistical Manual of Mental Disorders, Fourth Edition* (DSM-IV) criteria were utilized [4].

### Depression

Unipolar depression and dysthymia were evaluated according to DSM-IV criteria. Patient interviews, histories, psychiatric assessment forms, Beck Depression Inventory, and the PHQ-9 (Patient Health Questionnaire Depression Module) were utilized [4].

### The Bipolar Spectrum

Evaluation was accomplished by the following: (1) chart review, (2) Mood Disorder Questionnaire, (3) PHQ-9 (Patient Health Questionnaire Depression Module), and (4) interviews with patients and families.

The lifetime prevalence of bipolar, including the milder end of the spectrum, was assessed. Bipolar illness was defined according to the criteria established by the DSM-IV [4]. In addition, the modifications to DSM-IV by Akiskal were utilized in defining bipolar disorders [1, 74].

### Personality Disorders

The diagnosis of PD was done in accordance with DSM-IV criteria [4]. Patients with severe PDs were not placed on the opioids. Only patients deemed moderate to severe with PD psychopathology were included [78].

The PD characteristics were pervasive, longstanding, and influential in social and work functioning. The purpose of this was twofold: to identify patients at risk to themselves and their health care providers, and to exclude those with marginal PD diagnoses. Cluster A, B, and C PDs were included. The most prevalent were borderline, avoidant, dependent, and obsessive–compulsive.

### Attention Deficit Disorder

Patients with ADHD were included along with ADD. DSM-IV criteria were utilized [4]. Assessment was done via patient interviews, histories, and the Adult Self-Report Scale (ASRS).

### Exercise

Patients who exercised at least 20 min a day on average (140 min per week) were considered to be exercisers.

### Coping

Patients were assessed by the treating neurologist as to coping skills. Patients on disability due to headache were regarded as low copers. Medium to high copers were active and continued to work or go to school despite the presence of refractory pain.

### Working Patients

These patients continued to be employed 15 h per week or more, or worked full-time at home, with normal functioning.

### Disabled Patients

These patients were on long-term disability, or were unable to function more than minimally due to the CM.

### Fatigue

These patients had longstanding (greater than 6 months) chronic fatigue, or excessive daytime sleepiness. Other than the headache, fatigue and/or tiredness were a primary complaint.

### Statistical Analysis

Descriptive statistics (percentages) were used to summarize demographics and outcomes. A *Z*-test for proportion analysis was utilized. To be significant at the 0.05

level, the $Z$ had to be $> 1.96$. The $Z$-test was applied to groups with specific psychiatric diagnoses.

## *Results*

$n=115$ (87 female, 28 male, age range 23–77).

### Overall Efficacy and Number of Years on the Opioid

Sixty-five percent of patients were positive responders and response rates by type of patient or comorbid condition is summarized in Table 2.7. At the time of the study, the average number of years on the opioid for the positive responders was 4.5 years. The range was 9 months to 13 years. Seventy-three percent of patients reported at least one adverse event due to the opioid. The most common adverse events noted were: constipation (54 %), fatigue or somnolence (29 %), and nausea (21 %). Efficacy with regard to number of years of headache prior to starting the opioid was as follows:

- Three to fifteen years of headache prior to opioid: $n=37$, 69 % positive response.
- Sixteen or more years of headache prior to opioid: $n=78$, 61 % positive response.
- Overall rate of opioid abuse (as defined above) was $n=30/115$ (26 % of patients) as compared with previous abuse of SAOs, $n=32/115$ (28 %). Of the latter, 91 %

**Table 2.7** Summary of results by patient type or comorbidity (n/r=not reported)

| Group by patient type or comorbidity | % of total sample | % of group showing long-term positive results from opioids | % of group that qualified as opioid abusers |
|---|---|---|---|
| Anxiety (including generalized anxiety disorder, panic disorder, and obsessive–compulsive disorder) | 67/115 (58) | 44/67 (66) | 19/67 (28) |
| Depression (nonbipolar) | 76/115 (66) | 52/76 (68) | 21/76 (28) |
| Bipolar depression | 16/115 (14) | 10/16 (63) | 5/16 (31) |
| Personality disorders (PD) | 29/115 (25) | 10/29 (34) | 13/29 (45) |
| Attention deficit disorder (ADD) | 20/115 (17) | 13/20 (65) | 6/20 (30) |
| Exercisers | 43/115 (37) | 26/43 (60) | n/r |
| Nonexercisers | 72/115 (63) | 42/72 (58) | n/r |
| Low copers | 32/115 (27) | 16/32 (50) | 9/32 (28) |
| Medium to high copers | 83/115 (72) | 63/83 (76) | 21/83 (25) |
| Working patients | 75/115 (65) | 45/75 (60) | 20/75 (27) |
| Disabled patients | 19/115 (17) | 12/19 (63) | 4/19 (21) |
| Fatigue | 15/115 (13) | 10/15 (67) | n/r |

went on to abuse the LAOs as well. Information on smoking was available for 72 patients. Of the 53 identified nonsmokers, the abuse rate was 9/53 (17%) while for the 19 who had smoked at some point, the abuse rate was 4/19 (21%).

#### Statistical Analysis of Efficacy Rates

The rate of "positive efficacy" was compared to the rate of "no efficacy" for each of the following groups: those with anxiety, depression, bipolar depression, and PDs. A $Z$-test was utilized. To be significant at the 0.05 level, the $Z$ had to be $> 1.96$. There were no significant differences for any of the above diagnoses between those who had a "positive efficacy" outcome versus those with "no efficacy:"

> Patients with an increased chance of success included younger patients, high copers, and those without previous opioid abuse. Predicators of failure were those with personality disorders, older patients and, in particular, those with previous abuse of the short-acting opioids.

### *Discussion*

We assessed 115 patients with RCM who were treated with LAOs during a 6-year period. This was a select group of patients who had all done well previously with SAOs. All of the patients in this study had already been on SAOs for at least a year.

Sixty-five percent of the patients did well for at least 9 months on the opioid. The average duration of use of the opioid was 4.5 years. Forty-four percent of the patients reported adverse events. Patients with an increased chance of success included younger patients, high copers, and those without previous opioid abuse. Predicators of failure were those with PDs, older patients and, in particular, those with previous abuse of the SAOs. In this study, anxiety, depression, bipolar depression, ADD, exercise, working, disability, fatigue, or cigarette smoking did not significantly change the long-term outcome.

#### Previous Studies

In one of our previous studies conducted in 1999 [65], a significantly lower rate of success (13%) was obtained compared to the current study (65%). This was, in part, due to an altered standard of success utilized in the current study. The current study defined success as a 30% or more improvement in headache, compared to the 50% in the previous study. In addition, patient selection has been greatly improved. For this study, every patient selected had demonstrated a favorable response to SAOs. Also, while 29 of these 115 (25%) patients did have a PD, patients with severe PDs were not placed on opioids during this study period. This study ran from 2002 through 2007. I believe that our patient selection has steadily improved over the years, particularly in selecting those who have had success from SAOs without overuse and in not prescribing the opioids to those with severe PDs or other severe psychiatric problems.

In 1997, Saper and associates assessed refractory chronic daily headache with scheduled LAOs, particularly methadone [91]. There was a small subset of patients who did well. Similar results were obtained from Rothrock [87] and from Robbins [65]. Subsequently, Saper and his associates soured on the use of the opioids. An unpublished study from Rothrock indicated that in the CM patients who were responsive at 2 months to the methadone treatment, more than 70 % continued to maintain a response at 1 year [88]. Rothrock found that patients tend to either respond to relatively low doses or not respond at all. His studies also indicated that virtually all of the positive responders, when tapered off of the methadone, did relapse into their frequent headache patterns [88].

Saper found that only 10–15 % of initially enrolled patients experienced sustained, long-term, and meaningful improvement. Another meta-analysis of long-term efficacy with the opioids in more than 3000 patients resulted in the conclusion that there was no great evidence for sustained, long-term results in the majority of the patients [102]. In this, as in the majority of studies, there has been a high dropout rate due to adverse events and lack of pain relief.

Since 1870, opioids have gone through cycles of being overprescribed and underprescribed [36]. A balanced approach is probably best. Portenoy has stated that "There appears to be a select subpopulation of patients with chronic pain that can achieve sustained partial analgesia from opioid therapy without the occurrence of intolerable side effects or the development of aberrant drug-related behaviors [57]." In general, at least half of the patients who are prescribed opioids abandon them due to side effects or lack of efficacy.

Kalso analyzed 15 placebo-controlled studies involving 1145 patients for chronic, noncancer pain. Across all of the trials, the mean decrease in pain intensity was at least 30 % [38]. The vast majority (80 % of patients) suffered at least one adverse event. Constipation occurred in 41 % of patients, nausea in 32 %, and somnolence in 29 %. Fifty-six percent of the patients stopped the opioids due to lack of efficacy and/or side effects while 44 % continued in the long term. In various studies, the effects of opioids on QOL are inconsistent. Long-term, large, multicenter trials have not been done.

In one neurology office, Watson assessed 102 patients and concluded that opioids prescribed by the neurologist for chronic pain did lead to acceptable pain relief and decreased disability [108]. In a review of multiple randomized clinical trials, Farrar concluded that approximately a 30 % decrease in pain is the demarcation where most patients feel that it is relevant clinically [23]. Opioids have been tested versus tricyclic antidepressants (TCA) in several trials, and have generally proven somewhat more effective [102]. In one study in 2002, 54 % preferred the opioids versus 30 % the TCAs [59].

## SAOs Versus LAOs

Short acting generally refers to not only how long a drug carries the desired effect but also the speed of the onset of the drug and how fast it drops off toward the end of the dose. Quick onsets and fast drop-offs are major determinants for abuse [36]. SAOs are not necessarily quick-onset medications. Most oral SAO tablets are slow to take effect. A short duration of action then leads to frequent administration and overuse may occur. However, it has not been proven conclusively in studies that SAOs lead to less or more abuse or are more dangerous than LAOs.

In a previous study by Doley, 81 % of self-selected patients on SAOs had continued good efficacy with the same dose, averaging four tablets per day of 7.5 or 10 mg hydrocodone. Eighty-one percent did say that the opioid was just as effective as in the previous month, and stable dosing was noted in these patients for an average of 31 months. Seventy percent of the patients remained free of any overuse violations or infractions. In addition, the patients on the SAOs had an increased QOL [20]. Self-selected groups, such as in our current study here, will report better efficacy because all patients who were chosen did well on the SAOs.

Although certain drugs—such as oxycodone CR—are more easily abused, it is the person, not the drug, who governs abuse. While some abusers have only one drug of choice, many will tend to abuse a succession of drugs.

### Advantages and Disadvantages of LAOs

Several previous studies have evaluated daily opioids for severe chronic daily headache [63, 87, 91]. While success rates have been relatively low, they represent patients who have failed the usual ministrations, and who have few options available.

The advantages of LAOs include:

Avoidance of the "end-of-the-dose" phenomenon, with mini-withdrawals throughout the day
Consistent dosing one or two times daily, which decreases obsession with the next dose
Maintenance of stable blood levels
Avoidance of the acetaminophen, aspirin and NSAIDs that are included in many short-acting preparations
Probable diminished risk of significant abuse
Better compliance, with less psychological dependency on the drug

Disadvantages of LAOs include:

Social stigma
Fatigue and constipation
Difficulty in obtaining scripts, with no refills available
Need for frequent office visits and monitoring
Risk of OIH
Risk of abuse, although probably less than the SAOs
Interactions with other sedating drugs or alcohol
Risk of overdose

### LAOs and Abuse

Most opioid abuse is secondary to immediate-acting opioids or the longer-acting ones that are easily convertible to short-acting ones. An example of this would be oxycodone CR. Younger people, particularly older adolescents, are the most frequent abusers [110].

Since their introduction in 1982, the LAOs have not been shown to be widely abused. The transdermal fentanyl has been available since 1991, and has only been minimally abused. It does not have a quick onset of action. Oxycodone CR (Oxycontin) has greatly increased the abuse rate, possibly owing to its hydrophilic nature where crushing it leads to a very quick onset. The newer abuse-deterrent preparations have been of some (limited) help in curbing abuse. Most of the abuse of LAOs is ingesting multiple oral tablets, often along with alcohol. Crushing and snorting or shooting the opioids is not as prevalent as oral ingestion. Despite the inherent problems, there has been an increasing use of continuous slow-release preparations for chronic pain [2].

## *Definitions of Substance Use and Misuse*

### Physical Dependence

Physical dependence occurs with many drug classes, such as the SSRIs, nitroglycerin, and insulin, as well as opioids. This is an expected outcome of LAO use and is a normal physiologic consequence. It occurs within 3–10 days after initiation of the opioid, but the degree varies widely between patients. In physically dependent patients, the abstinence (withdrawal) syndrome will occur if the drug is suddenly discontinued. Unfortunately, physical dependence is too often confused with addiction.

### Opioid Abuse

Opioid abuse is much more common than true addiction. In general, using opioids for therapeutic reasons other than pain constitutes abuse. People who use opioids for mood enhancement are considered abusers. In a headache practice, the most common reasons for abuse are using the opioids to alleviate moods, anxiety, or depression.

Patients in the study were assessed for behaviors typical of opioid abuse or overuse as described earlier. There is a range of abuse, from the person who samples his spouse's codeine prescription once in a while to the addict who obtains hundreds of opioid tabs from the Internet. We should not paint all abusers with one broad brush. Some situations need watching, such as the patient who took her mom's pills because she had excess pain; this behavior is a red flag and the patient may be an abuser. For a different patient—for example, one who has already been prescribed low dose, long-acting morphine—the discovery of undisclosed opioid prescriptions from other sources must be regarded as severe abuse. In this situation, discontinuation of the opioids is necessary.

### Chemical Coping

In those who self-medicate, a drug is used for a purpose other than the intended one, such as using an opioid as a mood stabilizer or enhancer. Opioids can be both calming and stimulating, often giving a brief burst of energy and then a tranquil period. Chemical coping is all too common, but is poorly understood and under-researched [62]. All addicts are chemical copers to some degree, but not all people who cope chemically are addicts. The person who utilizes one or two pills of hydrocodone a day for stress and anxiety is not an addict by definition but is certainly using chemicals to cope. The severe chemical coping patients basically live for the drug; their lives are controlled by procurement of the drug, and they have few coping skills outside of using the drug [56]. They will self-escalate their drug use, particularly during periods of high stress. As much as 35 % of patients with chronic pain may fall under the definition of chemical copers [37]. There are gender differences, with women using the substances primarily for anxiety, stress, and depression. Women are at somewhat of an increased risk for chemically coping than are men [56].

Men may utilize the drugs for anxiety and depression, but also use them out of boredom and for sensation seeking. In particular, when men are disabled by their pain, they often chemically cope out of boredom. For some men, there is a strong relationship between substance abuse and sensation seeking [56].

### Tolerance

With opioid use, tolerance is a natural biological consequence. Tolerance means requiring increasing doses of the opioid in order to maintain the same response. Tolerance rates vary widely among patients, and younger people do develop tolerance more quickly than older individuals. As people age, their neurons lose some of the ability to develop tolerance. Many patients do not become tolerant to the analgesic effects and the same dose may be maintained for years. The tolerance to sedation is beneficial. Tolerance to constipation rarely occurs.

When tolerance to the analgesic effect does occur and the patient is at the upper limit of our comfort zone in prescribing, there are three options: adding a short-acting analgesic, switching opioids, or discontinuing opioids for a period of time. I believe it is a mistake to continuously increase the dose in the face of analgesic tolerance. For headache patients with nonmalignant chronic pain, I believe it is crucial to maintain low to medium doses of the opioid.

**Addiction**

While physical dependence and tolerance are to be expected with long-term opioid use, addiction is not. Addiction constitutes a biologic and behavioral disease. Most abusers can stop using the drug when harm occurs, but an addict cannot. Whether a patient with previous addictions should be treated with LAOs is a complicated issue. It should be approached on a case-by-case basis and is dependent on a number of factors. Among the considerations:

What substances were abused
How many years the patient has been clean
Whether the patient successfully completed treatment
The quality of the support system
Any comorbid psychiatric conditions [110]
Assessment of risk factors

Previous studies have indicated that risk factors for opioid abuse include the following: cigarette smoking, previous drug abuse, a strong family history of drug abuse, stress, young age, early sexual abuse, poor support, low level of functioning due to headache or other pain, pain embellishment, and certain psychiatric conditions [6, 22, 94]. Our current study affirms that those with PDs or previous abuse of short-term opioids are at an increased risk.

## *A Proposed Classification Scheme for Prescription Opioid Abuse*

It is too simplistic to view patients as "addicts versus nonaddicts." Dr. Sidney Schnoll, MD, PhD, has proposed a potentially useful classification system which describes subtypes of potential abusers. These include the following:

Health care professionals,
Illicit opioid addicts,
Prescription opioid addicts,
Polydrug abusers,
Rave abusers,
Casual abusers,
Patient abusers,
Patient diverters, and
Sham-patient diverters [39].

This scheme recognizes the variability among abusers; the subtypes represent differing levels and types of abuse. Many of our patient abusers may not be easily classified.

## *Screening for Abuse*

There are a number of diagnostic tools available for screening [13]. The Prescription Drug Use Questionnaire (PDUQ) is a long interview that is fairly predictive of substance abuse and liability. However, with 42 questions, it does take a fair amount of time. The shorter Opioid Risk Tool (ORT), with only five questions, has been validated as a simple initial screen [109]. The Screener and Opioid Assessment for Patients with Pain (SOAPP)® takes 10 min and is comprised of 24 items; a shorter, 14-question form is now available [9]. Each of these tools varies as far as sensitivity and specificity. While the SOAPT is highly sensitive (90 %) in picking up patients who will abuse the opioids, it also has a fairly high false-positive rate of about 30 % [8]. For patients new to a practice, assessment tools can quickly identify possible risks. However, risk assessment should be an ongoing process. Even for established patients, the screening tools are helpful. The best screen for abuse is a long and established relationship between the doctor and patient.

## *Specific Psychiatric Problems and Risk of Abuse*

An NIMH analysis identified certain problems that carried an increased risk for substance abuse. Of those with anxiety, 25 % had a substance use problem, as did 33 % of those with OCD and 61 % in the bipolar I category. Unipolar depression also carried a higher risk, but not as much as bipolar. Among PD patients, 84 % of those with antisocial PDs were substance abusers [7].

Untreated ADHD in older adolescent boys had a 75 % risk of substance abuse, while treated ADHD in this category falls to a 25 % risk. The boys without ADHD had an 18 % overall abuse rate [7]. Our study indicated that those with PDs were at an increased risk for abuse, but that other psychiatric conditions did not lead to more abuse.

Somatization is a complex syndrome, where the person has physical complaints with no demonstrable cause. Distress is turned into physical complaints. Somatizing patients are probably at an increased risk for opioid abuse. However, the risk of abuse in somatizing patients has not been adequately studied.

## *Guidelines for the Successful Management of LAOs in Headache Patients*

### Patient Selection

The patient has to be reliable, and well-known to the practitioner. Many of the problems occur with new patients. It is usually prudent to wait several visits before prescribing the LAOs and after the physician can establish that there has been little or no previous abuse. Also, the physician must have knowledge and experience in the use of these drugs.

Patients must have demonstrated an adequate response to SAOs. We prefer to restrict use of LAOs to patients who have received SAOs for 1 year or more. Of course, all of these patients will have been refractory to conventional, nonopioid therapies. The patient must truly be refractory to the usual ministrations, with multiple adequate trials of the usual preventive medications. In this author's view, previous abuse of opioids should exclude patients, inasmuch as the current study demonstrates that previous abuse of SAOs almost always leads to abuse of the LAOs. Pseudoaddiction is certainly encountered, but seems to be rare in headache patients. Be wary of the patient who claims he or she can tolerate almost no medications except for opioids.

The use of opioids in patients under 30 should be restricted. Younger patients are more likely to develop tolerance; the older patients, particularly after age 65–70, have lost the ability to do the "neuronal gymnastics" that are necessary in the development of tolerance. Therefore, older patients may remain on the same low dose for a number of years. If a younger patient fulfills all the requirements, such as truly being refractory, is psychologically normal, and at low risk for addiction, he or she may be the exception to the age rule. MOH should be ruled out.

Patients with characteristics of narcissistic, antisocial, borderline, histrionic, or paranoid PDs are at increased risk for abuse [85]. It is best to avoid opioids in these PD patients. Patients with avoidant or dependent PDs, however, may not be at an increased risk for these drugs. Note that there is a spectrum of severity with PD patients; those with a mild PD are at lower risk than those with a more severe PD.

It is also best to avoid the opioids in patients with severe axis I pathology, particularly severe depression and anxiety. Some of these patients may do well in the long term; however, the severe axis I pathology does raise the risk of abuse, although this has not been absolutely proven [91].

## The Multidisciplinary Approach

Management of those with CM involves a biopsychosocial approach. Patients must not rely simply on the drug in order to function. While medications may be a mainstay of therapy, other interventions must be employed. Active coping should be strongly encouraged with each visit and may involve a variety of approaches. These may include seeing a psychotherapist, physical therapist or other practitioner, or using self-help approaches such as exercise or biofeedback. Passive coping is a major predictor of disability in chronic pain patients. Beware of the patient who says, "Doctor, when you give me enough drugs to stop the pain, then I will go back to work." Those patients who rely only on opioids have less chance of sustaining long-term relief.

Mental health professionals are invaluable in caring for the severe pain patient and they can help in risk assessment. Physical therapy is a powerful tool that may help us minimize the use of drugs. Biofeedback has consistently proved helpful in motivated patients and chiropractic treatment, yoga, acupuncture, and massage are helpful for selected patients. Even though pharmacotherapy is the cornerstone of treatment, it is only part of a more comprehensive plan.

### Three Phases of Treatment

There are three distinct phases in the use of opioids. The first phase is the initiation of treatment. This includes the initial screening and risk assessment, the doctor's decision as to which opioid to utilize, and the doctor–patient discussion and signing of an opioid agreement. Prior to initiation of LAOs, an assessment of the following should be done: pain level, moods, social and family functioning, work status, physical functioning, and activities of daily living [23].

The intermediate phase comprises the diligent monitoring of the patient while on the opioid. This must include ongoing assessment of the patient's pain level and overall functioning, with a watchful eye for signs of abuse. If patients do not report an improvement in functioning, or if functioning declines, consideration should be given for withdrawal from the opioid. Some patients have an improvement in pain but a decline in activity, possibly due to sedation or other opioid-related side effects.

The third phase is switching or withdrawing the opioids when abuse has occurred, or there is lack of efficacy. Withdrawing or switching an opioid may be exceedingly difficult in some patients. Each of these phases involves a learning curve on the part of the practitioner, and proper documentation by staff members.

The guidelines for initiation and maintenance of the opioids cannot be absolute, as that would inhibit the utilization of these drugs in appropriate patients. Requiring that every patient has multiple visits with the prescribing physician, sees a primary care doctor, and consults a psychologist prior to administration of the opioids is simply not practical. The above steps are helpful and necessary for certain patients but, in others, opioids may be initiated using less rigid guidelines. We do not want to make the requirements for the initiation and maintenance of opioids so onerous as to render them impractical. Note this is an updated version of an article that originally appeared in *Practical Pain Management,* Issue 6, July 2009.

It is helpful to involve family members or significant others, other health care practitioners, and to review previous medical records. Spouses or other significant people in the patient's life often give a more accurate depiction of functioning and moods than the patient himself can. Speaking with the other health practitioners who are involved with the patient, and reviewing previous medical records may be invaluable in assessing the appropriateness of the opioids and the risk for abuse.

### Dosing and Titration for Migraineurs

In my experience with migraineurs, higher doses of the opioid rarely work out in the long term. They place the patient at an increased risk of addiction and abuse, and complications from withdrawal. It may be thought that, given the great variation in individual responses, the opioid should be increased or "pushed" to whatever level is beneficial. However, medical and regulatory considerations should be limiting factors in keeping the opioid dose at a low level. The choice of opioid may be key; some have been shown to have less abuse potential. The long-acting fentanyl patch is subject to less abuse than oxycodone CR. The once- or twice-daily, long-acting morphine preparations have not been subjected to widespread abuse.

Methadone may be more effective than some of the other medications, but has a litany of problems associated with it. Besides the social stigma, high protein binding is a risk which may lead to irregular drug levels, difficulty with withdrawal, and an increased risk for sudden death [64]. If methadone is used, it should be started at a very low dose of no more than 5–10 mg a day, and titrated slowly. Patients placed on methadone require close monitoring, and other sedatives must be reduced or discontinued.

The usual dosing range for LAOs in my practice is:

Methadone, 5–40 mg per day
Hydrocodone, 15–50 mg per day
Morphine, 20–90 mg per day
Oxycodone, 20–60 mg per day
Buprenorphine patch, 10–20 mg per day

## The Opioid Agreement

Some type of written opioid agreement should be part of the doctorpatient alliance, although there is a lack of evidence that these agreements do much good for the majority of the patients. There is no standard opioid contract; practices should adapt one for their own purposes.

An agreement sets limits, educates the patient, deals with patient responsibilities, discusses termination criteria, and should include mention of urine testing for drugs. It is a bilateral agreement; the physician can be held accountable for its contents. For instance, there was a case where the patient violated the agreement, yet the physician continued to prescribe. When the patient overdosed and died, the physician was held liable in court [12].

Probably the best evidence of the benefits of the opioid agreement is seen in patients with known addiction histories. The agreement in this situation may improve compliance. Considerations for the agreement should include the following:

Do not label it as a contract, but rather as a patient–physician agreement.
Carefully word the agreement so as to minimize risk to the physician.
Do not word it punitively toward the patient.
Use the agreement primarily as education and to outline limits.
Consider having the patients' primary care physician also sign the agreement.

There are several resources on opioid agreements, such as the American Association of Physicists in Medicine (AAPM) website, www.painmed.org; the American

Pain Society website, www.ampainsoc.org; the Federation of State Medical Boards, Inc., www.fsmb.org; and the US Drug Enforcement Administration (DEA), www.usdoj.gov/dea. In addition, there is an excellent article on agreement contracts by Fishman [25].

### Ongoing Assessment

Every visit after the initial one should include an assessment of function, mood, pain level, abuse, adverse events, and a brief physical exam. The physical exam on a return visit needs to primarily assess for slurring of words, abnormal gait, and pupillary abnormalities. Patients usually respond fairly quickly to an opioid. If they have not responded by 2–4 weeks of a low dose, there usually will not be an adequate response [88]. With no or little response by 4 weeks, the consideration should be for switching or discontinuing the opioid.

### Urine Testing

Do not assume that low-risk patients will never abuse the opioids. During the maintenance phase of opioid prescribing, it is remarkable how many seemingly low-risk patients do misuse the drugs.

There are two purposes to testing. One is to identify other substances that may be present though they should not be. Another is to detect the levels of the prescribed substance for compliance. When there is no opioid present, there is sometimes a laboratory error or test insensitivity, but it possible that the patient has been binging early on and has run out of drugs before the visit [30]. Another possibility is that the patient is selling the drugs.

In my experience, the pain patients who raise objections and do not grant urine test requests usually have a drug problem. Specimen collections should be random and not scheduled. Most of the illegal drugs and metabolites last in the urine for 1–3 days [106]. Urine panel screens should include cocaine, amphetamines, opioids, methadone, tetrahydrocannabinol (THC), and benzodiazepines. Immunoassay urine screening is simple and has high sensitivity but lacks specificity. Chromatographic testing is better [10]. Combined testing techniques, such as gas chromatography/mass spectrometry (GC/MS), are even more accurate.

### Breakthrough Pain

The treatment of breakthrough pain is controversial. Most of the breakthrough studies have been concerned with cancer pain where the average number of breakthroughs is 4 per 24 h [111]. For patients with noncancer breakthrough pain, such as chronic daily headache, I tend to minimize the total opioid and avoid layering pain medicines on top of each other. Prescribing short-acting medications, such as hydrocodone, for chronic headaches greatly increases the abuse rate. The occasional patient can remain on a low dose of the LAO, with one or two SAOs such as hydrocodone per day but, in general, try to avoid these SAOs.

## When Tolerance Occurs

There are three components to tolerance: pharmacologic tolerance, OIH, and increased pain due to disease progression. While the last usually refers to cancer-type pain, it may also occur with the headache patient. OIH occurs where the opioid facilitates nociceptive events; this counteracts the positive results from the opioid medication [48]. When patients become tolerant to the positive effect of the opioids, a switch in opioids may be more beneficial than increasing the dose. Cross-tolerance of opioids is often incomplete, so that rotating the opioids may be of benefit. To change opioids, we generally start at 40–70 % of the equivalent dose of the old medication. Actively managing the accompanying constipation is crucial in order to improve compliance:

> With careful patient selection and close monitoring, certain patients may do well for many years on opioids and may significantly improve pain and quality of life.

Heed red flags! If a relatively new patient calls with a tale such as, "the tablets fell down the sink," we need to be careful about giving the patient the benefit of the doubt. How often are stories like this true? Of course, a situation from a long-term patient who has never shown signs of abuse may be more believable than a new patient with the same story.

It is not always clear how serious the abuse is. The discovery that a patient received six tablets of hydrocodone from a dentist is probably innocuous, although it would be better if the patient had informed your office. However, finding that a patient that you have on morphine is also receiving 30 tablets of hydrocodone from an internist warrants serious consideration for discontinuation.

Minor aberrant behaviors are often overlooked. It is not as if any one aberrant behavior warrants immediate discontinuation of an opioid, but most of the serious overuse situations have previously had a number of minor abuse occurrences. Physicians must pay attention to red flags, particularly those that arise early in the relationship with the patient.

A number of national organizations have published guidelines and standards for opioid prescribing. The consensus is that opioids are appropriate for certain legitimate pain patients, but the practitioner needs to observe state and federal guidelines. More information is available through their websites, including: American Pain Society, www.ampainsoc.org; American Society of Addiction Medicine, www.asam.org; American Academy of Pain Medicine, www.painmed.org; American Academy of Pain Management, www.aapainmanage.org. The excellent site www.legalsideofpain.com is a terrific source for the practitioner.

## *Conclusion*

CM remains undertreated, as only approximately 50 % of patients do well in the long term with preventatives. The other half remains at a loss. Untreated, chronic pain has an enormous impact on a patient's economic situation and QOL. When these patients are successfully treated, many will demonstrate significant functional improvement. With careful patient selection and close monitoring, certain patients may do well for many years on opioids and may significantly improve pain and QOL.

Patient selection is key, and monitoring of opioid use must be continual and vigilant. While use of opioids does carry risks for migraineurs, all of the other medication choices for these refractory patients have side effects. Patients more likely to do well include younger patients, high copers, and those without previous opioid abuse. Predictors of failure are older patients, PDs and, in particular, those who previously abused opioids. Patients with anxiety, depression, bipolar disorder, or ADD did as well as those without these comorbidities. Cigarette smoking was not a predictor for abuse. For a limited number of carefully selected patients who are not opioid-naive LAOs may be a successful option. Note this is an updated version of an article that originally appeared in *Practical Pain Management*.

# Stimulant Use in Migraineurs

> Stimulants may be beneficial for chronic migraine patients presenting with various comorbidities such as attention deficit hyperactivity disorder (ADHD), depression and fatigue.

Amphetamines have been shown to possess intrinsic analgesic properties, primarily through brain catecholamine activity. They also intensify the analgesic effects of certain opioids [21]. When prescribed for headache patients, stimulants may be beneficial for various comorbidities such as ADHD, depression, and fatigue. In addition, stimulants do not cause the weight gain that is seen with a number of other current headache preventives.

This chapter reviews our experience with stimulants in CM patients over a period of 6 years.

## *Methods*

### Study Design

This retrospective study was conducted at a single US headache clinic. Data were collected via chart review, patient diary, and patient interview. Patients who had been prescribed stimulants during the 6-year period of 2002–2007 were assessed.

Patients kept a headache diary and used a ten-point visual analog scale to measure the severity of the pain.

Patient Characteristics: Seventy-three patients (57 female, 16 male) were evaluated. The patients had been diagnosed previously as having CM. With a few exceptions, the stimulants were prescribed primarily for the associated comorbidities. The comorbidities (some patients had more than one) included: ADHD ($n$=28), unipolar depression ($n$=28), fatigue/sleepiness ($n$=17), bipolar depression ($n$=14), and narcolepsy ($n$=3).

Inclusion Criteria: Long-time patients at the treating headache clinic with the diagnosis of CM were included. CM was defined according to the International Headache Society criteria [100]. All patients had been prescribed stimulants, including amphetamine/ dextroamphetamine, dextroamphetamine, and methylphenidate.

Primary Outcome Measure: The primary outcome measure was efficacy of the stimulant with regard to headache. Efficacy was determined to be positive if the patient continued on the stimulant for at least 9 months and consistently reported a 30% or more improvement in headache frequency and/or severity over a 3-month baseline.

## Results

Efficacy: Of the 73 patients, 55 (75%) continued on the stimulant for at least 9 months. Of the 55 patients, 26 (47%) met the standard of efficacy of at least a 30% decrease in headache frequency and/or severity. Of the original 73 patients, 34% remained on the stimulant and reported positive headache efficacy.

Efficacy in Relation to Comorbidity: The positive headache response allocated by comorbidity is presented in Table 2.8.

Adverse Events: Of 73, 30 (41%) of the patients experienced at least one side effect. The side effects are presented in Table 2.9 (note that some patients reported multiple side effects).

Abuse or addiction: Two patients (3%) abused the stimulant.

## Discussion

Psychopharmacology of Stimulants: Common stimulants include nicotine, caffeine, amphetamine, and amphetamine derivatives. As a group, CNS stimulants cause

**Table 2.8** Efficacy in relation to comorbidity

| Comorbidity | No. of patients with comorbidity | No. of patients with positive efficacy | % of patients with positive efficacy |
|---|---|---|---|
| ADHD | 28 | 7 | 25 |
| Unipolar depression | 28 | 8 | 29 |
| Fatigue/sleepiness | 17 | 6 | 35 |
| Bipolar depression | 14 | 3 | 21 |
| Narcolepsy | 3 | 2 | 66 |

*ADHD* attention-deficit hyperactivity disorder

**Table 2.9** Summary of adverse events

| Side effect | No | % |
|---|---|---|
| Anxiety | 9 | 12 |
| Increased headache | 9 | 12 |
| Insomnia | 7 | 10 |
| Decreased appetite | 6 | 8 |
| Nausea | 6 | 8 |
| Dry mouth | 5 | 7 |
| Tachycardia | 4 | 5 |
| Depression | 4 | 5 |
| Hypertension | 2 | 3 |
| Diarrhea | 2 | 3 |

excitement and euphoria, decrease feelings of fatigue, and increase motor activity [24]. Caffeine, the most widely consumed stimulant in the world, is believed to act by several mechanisms of action in the prefrontal cortex and other areas of the brain. These include translocation of extracellular calcium, inhibition of phosphodiesterase and adenosine receptor antagonism, resulting in decreased fatigue and increased mental alertness [24].

Nicotine, the active ingredient in tobacco, specifically stimulates nicotinic receptors in the autonomic ganglia, resulting in euphoria, arousal, relaxation, improved attention, learning, problem solving, and reaction time [24]. However, in very high doses, nicotine causes blockade of autonomic ganglia, resulting in respiratory depression and severe hypotension.

Cocaine acts to stimulate the CNS in a more indirect manner by blocking reuptake of norepinephrine, serotonin, and dopamine into the presynaptic terminal from which they are released [24]. This reuptake antagonism serves to potentiate and prolong the CNS and PNS effects of these catecholamines. In the CNS, this results in intense euphoria, acutely increased mental awareness and increased motor activity. At high doses, these effects manifest as hallucinations, delusions, paranoia, tremors, and convulsions. Peripherally, the effects of cocaine include tachycardia, hypertension, pupillary dilation, and peripheral vasoconstriction [24].

Amphetamine and its derivatives, such as methylphenidate, demonstrate indirect CNS and PNS effects similar to cocaine. Like cocaine, they initially increase levels of catecholamines. However, amphetamines do this by a different mechanism of action. They accomplish this effect by causing the release of intracellular stores of catecholamines and inhibiting MAO [24]. The major cause of the behavioral effects of amphetamines is thought to be due more to release of dopamine rather than norepinephrine [24]. This ultimately results in increased alertness, decreased fatigue, decreased appetite and insomnia, as well as the usual "fight or flight" response characteristic of adrenergic stimulation in the PNS.

Stimulants and Headache: Our study assessed 73 chronic migraineurs who had been prescribed stimulants in addition to their other medications. While the stimulants were primarily prescribed for certain comorbidities, their effect on headaches was also assessed. Seventy-five percent of the patients placed on the stimulants remained on them for at least 9 months. Thirty-four percent of the 73 patients both remained on the stimulants and reported positive efficacy with regard to headache. Forty-one percent of the patients suffered at least one adverse event, while only two patients abused the stimulant.

Amphetamines have been known to possess independent analgesic activity, possibly due to release of norepinephrine. The effect was felt to be about the same as that of ibuprofen. Also, stimulants may potentiate the analgesic actions of opioids [17]. The most commonly studied combination has been dextroamphetamine and morphine. Methylphenidate has also been studied as an opioid adjunctive medication.

In one small study, the use of dextroamphetamine for patients with tension and migraine headache was assessed. It concluded that dextroamphetamine was viable as a preventive medication for chronic tension and migraine headaches in some subjects [32]. In another case report, a man was successfully treated with methylphenidate for his refractory episodic cluster headaches [52].

Stimulants have been utilized to counteract the sedation encountered by opioids. An excellent review article on stimulants as adjuncts for opioids concluded that, "The evidence suggests that amphetamine drugs may enhance the effect of opioids and, at the same time, decrease somnolence and increase cognitive performance [17]."

Which headache patients should receive stimulants? Those with ADHD certainly warrant consideration. For refractory headache, where little has helped, occasionally stimulants help both pain and energy. Many of our patients are overweight and tired, with poor concentration, and stimulants may help these comorbidities. Stimulants are occasionally helpful for depression, as adjunctive medication. By themselves they are not very effective antidepressants. Keeping doses low is a key. Many patients do well for months or years, as long as they are able to stick to lower doses of stimulants.

## *Conclusion*

Stimulants have proven utility for certain conditions such as ADHD. This study demonstrates that for patients with these comorbidities, the stimulants may also be beneficial for a minority of patients with CM.

Advantages of stimulants include enhanced cognition and alertness but with no weight gain. Disadvantages primarily revolve around the side effects, such as anxiety or insomnia. Abuse may certainly occur but it is uncommon in adults. Stimulants should be considered in patients with certain comorbidities. The few studies to date have indicated a positive role for stimulants but further studies on stimulants for headache would help to clarify that role. Note this is an updated version of an article originally published in *Practical Pain Management,* Vol. 9, Sept. 2009.

## Brief Communication

### *Frequent Triptan Use: Observations on Safety Issues*

L. Robbins MD

Note this article was previously published in *Headache* (2004).

Objective: To examine the safety of frequent triptan use over extended periods. For a small group of patients with refractory migraine plus chronic daily headache, triptans are effective.
Methods: This retrospective study primarily evaluated the cardiac safety of daily triptan use in 118 patients and, in addition, hematologic tests were assessed. Each patient had utilized a triptan for a minimum of 4 days per week for at least 6 months. Patients with rebound headache had been withdrawn from the triptans. Most patients (97 of 118) averaged one tablet daily; most would occasionally go for several days without a triptan. Forty patients had taken a triptan for 6 months to 2 years, 37 patients from 2 to 4 years, and 41 for 4 or more years.
Results: Routine hematologic tests were performed periodically on all patients, and no abnormalities were attributable to triptans. Almost all patients had an electrocardiogram (ECG), and no abnormal ECGs were felt to be related to triptans. Cardiac echocardiography was performed in 57 patients. The ten abnormal echocardiograms were not due to triptans. All 20 cardiac stress tests revealed normal findings. Adverse events were minimal; nine patients described fatigue due to triptans, and five had mild chest tightness.
Conclusion: This long-term study of 118 patients indicates that frequent triptan use may be relatively safe.
Keywords: triptan, chronic daily headache, migraine
Abbreviations: CDH chronic daily headache
(*Headache* 2004;44:178–182)

Many patients' migraine and chronic daily headache (CDH) are refractory to the usual preventive medications. One previous study of patients with CDH indicated that, over the long term, only 46 % would respond to preventives [83]. The usual preventives include: antidepressants, anticonvulsants, beta-adrenergic blocking agents, calcium channel antagonists, and muscle relaxants [68]. For those who continue to experience moderate or severe headache on a frequent basis, medication choices are limited. These include (among others) opioids [63], monoamine oxidase inhibitors (MAOIs) [19], botulinum toxin injections [29], or a combination of preventives.

Some patients respond only to triptan medications (sumatriptan, naratriptan, rizatriptan, almotriptan, zolmitriptan, frovatriptan, eletriptan). Several studies have described the use of daily triptans for the preventive treatment of CDH [61, 84, 98]. The patients in this study were never instructed to use triptans on a daily basis. They "self-discovered" that a dose of triptan would alleviate headache for most or all of the day. Most patients in this study had a long history of headache refractory to usual medications. They finally had found a medication (a triptan) that would alleviate the headache for some time.

Most of the patients had been using frequent triptans through their primary care physician. A minority of our patients had increased the amount of triptan prescribed. Patients were withdrawn from triptans in order to determine if rebound headache was present. The only patients who continued on triptans were those who: (1) had been determined to truly be refractory to other approaches, (2) experienced no or minimal side effects, (3) had rebound headaches excluded, and (4) signed a

"Frequent Triptan Informed Consent" form. Many patients did not meet these criterion, and the triptans were discontinued.

One goal of this retrospective study of a large group of patients was to evaluate the cardiac safety of triptans. A secondary objective was to assess the hematologic tests that were performed in these patients.

## *Patients and Methods*

### Patients

A total of 118 patients (27 men and 91 women), aged 27–73 years (mean, 52), were evaluated. Inclusion criteria were: (1) the patient had used a triptan for a minimum of 4 days weekly, for at least 6 months and (2) all patients would occasionally go days without a triptan. Exclusion criteria included: (1) the presence of rebound headache (patients were withdrawn from the triptan before 6 months), (2) not utilizing a triptan at least 4 days weekly on a consistent basis, and (3) had not had adequate trials of standard preventive approaches. All patients had signed a "Frequent Triptan Informed Consent" form.

### Previous Medications

All study participants were long-term patients at the Robbins Headache Clinic. Each patient's headache had been refractory to at least three of the usual preventive medications. These included: beta-adrenergic blocking agents, calcium channel antagonists, antidepressants, anticonvulsants, methysergide, nonsteroidal anti-inflammatory drugs (NSAIDs, and muscle relaxants. Most patients' headaches had been refractory to five or more daily preventives. During the study, besides the triptan, most patients continued on at least one preventive medication, the most common of which were antidepressants. Some patients also used NSAIDs or other analgesics.

### Rebound Headache

Patients were carefully screened for the presence of rebound headache. If the history was possibly consistent with rebound headache, the patient was withdrawn from the triptan. All patients were withdrawn from the triptan for a period, to help exclude the possibility of rebound headache.

### Patient Assessment

The treating neurologist at Robbins Headache Clinic performed the interviews and chart reviews. Hematologic, electrocardiographic, and echocardiographic findings were assessed via retrospective chart reviews. In patients on daily triptans, as a matter of routine (at this clinic), hematologic tests were regularly done, as were ECGs. Cardiac echocardiography with Doppler flow studies was accomplished in 57 (almost half) patients.

### Type of Headache

Headache classification was based on International Headache Society (IHS) revisions proposed by Silberstein et al. [99]. Of 118 patients, 107 were diagnosed with migraine plus CDH, 2 patients with CDH alone, and 9 patients had chronic cluster headache.

### Type of Triptan

During the course of treatment, most patients switched from one triptan to another, and often reverted to the original one. Reasons for this included tolerance and insurance issues.

Patients had taken the stated triptan for at least 2 months: 85 patients used sumatriptan, 68 naratriptan, 37 rizatriptan, 30 zolmitriptan, and 6 almotriptan.

### Amount of Triptan

For most of the treatment course, most patients (97 of 118) averaged one tablet daily (50 mg sumatriptan, 2.5 mg naratriptan, 10 mg rizatriptan, 5 mg zolmitriptan). Eight patients used only half a tablet daily, while eight used 0.5 tablets on a daily basis. Five patients consumed two tablets daily. Ninety patients used the triptan every day, while 28 patients averaged 4–5 days per week. All of the patients would occasionally go for several days without a triptan (or occasionally take a drug holiday for weeks).

Forty patients had taken a triptan for 6 months to 2 years, 37 for 2–4 years, 29 for 4–6 years, and 12 patients took a triptan for more than 6 years. Forty-one patients had taken daily triptans for 4 or more years (Table 2.10).

## *Results*

### Laboratory (Hematologic) Tests

Routine blood tests including complete blood counts and complete chemistries (liver and kidney functions, as well as cholesterol levels) were performed regularly, usually every 6–9 months, on all patients. Thirty-two patients had an increased cholesterol level, 12 patients had increased liver enzymes, and 3 had anemia. Two

**Table 2.10** Duration of triptan use in study participants

| Triptan use, no. of months | No. (%) of patients ($n$=118) |
|---|---|
| 6–12 | 18 (15) |
| 13–18 | 9 (8) |
| 19–24 | 13 (11) |
| 25–30 | 9 (8) |
| 31–36 | 11 (9) |
| 37–42 | 11 (9) |
| 43–47 | 6 (5) |
| 48–53 | 10 (8) |
| 54–60 | 9 (8) |
| 61–66 | 3 (3) |
| 67–72 | 7 (6) |
| 73–78 | 12 (10) |

patients had an increased blood urea nitrogen, and 1 had a decrease in platelets. None of the laboratory abnormalities were felt to be due to triptans.

### Cardiac Stress Test

Twenty patients had cardiac stress tests; all were normal. The stress tests were done for various reasons, unrelated to the triptans. One patient had a cardiac catheterization which was normal.

### Adverse Events

Nine patients felt that the triptans contributed to fatigue. Five patients had mild chest tightness, at times, possibly due to the triptans cardiac disease was ruled out. Three patients felt that the triptans contributed to nausea. Because these patients decided on their own to use triptans on a daily basis, adverse events would be expected to be low. If patients were not tolerating the medication well or were having significant adverse effects, they would not choose to continue the triptan on a frequent basis.

### Electrocardiograms

The study participants were not at high risk for cardiac disease; the ECGs were performed prospectively due to the nature of the medication, after a minimum of 6 months of daily triptan use. Most patients had an ECG during 2001 or 2002, which was toward the end of the study. A cardiologist evaluated the ECGs. No abnormalities were felt to be related to triptans. One hundred three patients had an ECG, 95 tracings were normal. The following abnormal ECG findings were apparent in eight patients: atrial fibrillation, $n$=1; tachycardia, $n$=2; bradycardia, $n$=1; inverted T waves, $n=1$; nonspecific ST-T wave changes, $n=2$; and rare premature atrial contractions, $n=1$.

#### Echocardiogram with Doppler

Fifty-seven patients underwent echocardiography with Doppler flow studies. The echocardiograms were performed a minimum of 9 months after the onset of daily triptan use to screen for cardiac abnormalities that may have occurred during the course of treatment. Most patients had an echocardiogram during the past 1.5 years of the study.

The attending cardiologist or internist saw the ten patients with an abnormal echocardiogram. None of the abnormalities were felt to be due to use of triptans. Six patients had mitral valve prolapse, and mitral regurgitation, enlarged aorta, mild right ventral enlargement, and aortic regurgitation were each found in one patient.

### *Comments*

In this current study, there were no adverse consequences from frequent use of triptans over a prolonged period. A total of 118 patients (primarily with migraine plus CDH) had "self-selected" triptans as the only beneficial treatment for their daily headaches. These patients had been refractory to the usual CDH and migraine preventives.

ECG, echocardiography with Doppler, and laboratory blood tests were performed. There may be adverse consequences of daily triptan use that were not detected in this study.

Our previous study assessed 59 patients with migraine plus CDH [84]. As in the current study, the patients had taken a daily (or near-daily) dose of a triptan for a minimum of 6 months. These patients had found daily triptans to be beneficial after years of failing various preventive regimens.

In our previous study, 23 patients (39 %) had been on triptans for 6–12 months, while 36 (61 %) had been on them for more than 1 year [84]. The patients had previously failed multiple first- and second-line preventive medications. Forty-one patients (69 %) were currently on preventive medications, the most common being sodium valproate and antidepressants. Forty-five patients (76 %) used abortive medications, in addition to the daily triptans. While 39 patients (66 %) had previously overused abortives, they were not overusing them since being on daily triptans. Side effects were minimal in this patient population. As in the current study, however, since the patients self-selected daily triptan use, side effects would be expected to be low. All patients had been carefully screened for rebound headache. Blood tests were done on all patients. Results were within the reference range in 47 of the 59 patients. None of the abnormal test results were felt to be due to triptans. ECGs revealed normal tracings in 19 of the 23 patients who had this procedure, while

4 patients had abnormal findings. The abnormal ECG results were not felt to be due to triptans. Echocardiography was done on five patients with no abnormalities [84].

Short-lasting adverse events are often encountered with triptan use. These include paresthesias, fatigue, chest heaviness, jaw or neck discomfort, etc. [46, 107].

Chest symptoms are, with rare exceptions, not of cardiovascular origin. Cardiac ischemia due to triptan use is rare [15, 104]. Triptans do constrict coronary vessels, but this is a mild and short-lived effect. Despite widespread triptan use, the number of adverse cardiac events has been limited [103]. Echocardiography and electrocardio graphy generally have been normal after triptan use, even in the presence of chest symptoms [16, 35].

The primary issue with frequent triptan use, assuming rebound headache is not present, is long-term adverse events. The cardiovascular system would be the most likely for possible long-term sequelae. Chronic ischemic changes, valvular abnormalities, or fibrosis are theoretical considerations. To date, there is no evidence of long-term frequent triptan use producing any of these adverse events. This has not been systematically studied, however. The number of patients throughout the world who have utilized near-daily triptans is unknown. Until these patients have been studied, it is reasonable and prudent to do cardiac monitoring, as well as hematologic tests.

While adverse effects from long-term triptan use are unknown, the alternatives have potential problems. Many patients with CDH are overusing analgesics, which have well-known adverse events [50]. These include liver dysfunction, gastrointestinal bleeding, renal insufficiency, and addiction.

Many patients' headaches have been refractory to daily preventive medications. The use of frequent triptans may help a limited number of these patients. We will need further studies to evaluate the safety of frequent triptan use. Note this originally appeared in *Headache,* Vol. 44, 2004.

## Migraine Headache Surgery (Letter; February, 2014 Headache)

The excellent article by Mathew, "A Critical Evaluation of Migraine Trigger Site Deactivation Surgery," casts doubt on the data supporting migraine surgery [31, 49]. Migraine surgery is being promoted by plastic surgeons. A common statement on certain surgery sites states that "of the 60–80 % of patients who respond to Botox, 90 % will benefit from migraine surgery." The word "cure" appears all too often.

The following are observations about migraine surgery:

1. Migraine is a complex syndrome involving genetics, brain chemistry, neuroinflammation, behavioral aspects, etc., and it is unlikely that a simple surgery would fix all of these factors.
2. Response to Botox (which most of the surgeons use as a guideline) should not necessarily predict a successful surgery; the mechanism of action of Botox

for migraines probably involves, among other factors, an anti-inflammatory response, not simply via muscle relaxation.

3. The surgery is supposed to be primarily for refractory migraine patients but is being done for those with new onset daily persistent headache (NDPH), post-traumatic headache, occipital neuralgia, and other varied headache syndromes.
4. Migraine and NDPH patients who have not had trials of medications are being operated upon, some of whom have had headaches for less than 1 year, and the patients have not necessarily been under the care of a neurologist or headache specialist.
5. Surgery about the head is not new: migraine patients who have undergone various cosmetic procedures (which are similar to the surgery being promoted) have not reported (in my experience) an improvement in headaches.
6. The disappointment after failed surgery cannot be underestimated. A young man in my practice had NDPH and was 50 % improved over 6 months. We could not dissuade him from undergoing the surgery (he was enthralled by the website claims), and after the surgery failed, this patient committed suicide. He was severely depressed, but the disappointment may have been a contributing factor.
7. Adverse events from the surgery should not be minimized; these are sensitized patients, often with allodynia, and cutting structures about the headache may lead to increased headaches or new neuralgia pains.
8. My "anecdotal scorecard" for the surgery results in about a 10 % success rate, not the 90 % often stated on the surgery websites.
9. We need multicenter trials to evaluate migraine surgery. Without adequate studies, the surgery remains an unproven and experimental procedure. Note this letter originally appeared in *Headache*, Vol. 54, Feb. 2014.

## In Defense of Butalbital

The article on butalbital-containing medicines (BCMs) by Tfelt-Hansen and Diener [105] accurately summarizes the literature. They appropriately call for a limit on BCM. However, the authors oversimplify an important and complex topic. There are significant advantages to BCM that should also be acknowledged.

Why use BCM? We use BCM partly because our alternatives often fall short. Triptans and dihydroergotamine do not work for many patients, may not be appropriate for others, or may be limited because of finances and insurance. Many patients take their triptan, and later, they also utilize an analgesic, such as a BCM. Ergots are rarely appropriate. Nonsteroidal anti-inflammatory drugs and aspirin are only mildly effective and have significant side effects, particularly with advancing age. Over-the-counter combinations (usually containing caffeine) are only modestly effective. They may cause MOH and may cause other adverse effects. Isometheptene-containing compounds have limited efficacy, may not be well-tolerated, and often are unavailable. Opioids create the same problems as BCM, with overuse, addiction, and adverse effects being commonplace.

To minimize the use of BCM (and other abortives), preventives are utilized. However, the available preventives often fail over the long term [69]. Previously, I evaluated preventives in 540 chronic headache patients over a 6-month time period. Only 46 % of patients remained on any preventive for at least 6 months. Fifty-four percent of patients dropped off of the preventives because of declining efficacy and/ or adverse reactions [83].

The use of onabotulinumtoxinA (Botox) has improved our success with preventives. Many patients, however, cannot afford the injections or find that the Botox is ineffective. Even those who do find some success with preventives still require abortive medications, such as BCM.

The positive attributes of BCM include: (1) reasonable efficacy (primarily anecdotal); (2) low cost; (3) minimal cardiac and other side effects (except for sedation); (4) relatively few drug interactions, they may be used with most other abortives, such as triptans; (5) reasonably well-tolerated at older age ranges; (6) versatility, available with acetaminophen or aspirin, with or without caffeine, and with or without codeine; (7) BCM may alleviate both migraine and tension-type headaches; (8) antianxiety effects (though we would not specifically prescribe BCM to treat anxiety or moods); (9) BCM will produce a mild euphoria or act as a mood enhancer in some individuals; while this is not our intent on prescribing BCM, in certain patients, this is not an undesirable side effect, improving QOL; (10) in some patients, BCM will alleviate certain other painful conditions, such as fibromyalgia, neck or back pain, or arthritis; while we would not specifically prescribe BCM for those conditions, the relief of other painful conditions may enhance QOL; and (11) refractory headache patients usually require analgesics, and BCMs are one of our available choices [82].

The downsides of BCM include the milder side effects (such as fatigue), the tendency of these drugs to contribute to MOH, and most importantly, the risk of addiction. Medication overuse (MO) is common among those with CM, but MO does not always lead to MOH. BCM, along with opioids and high-caffeine-containing analgesics, are more likely to cause MOH than most abortives, such as triptans. Dependence upon BCM is occasionally encountered, with the dose remaining stable for months or years. Dependence may be justified in some patients with chronic pain. True addiction also occurs with the use of BCM, where patients cross the line into a set of addictive behaviors. Addiction and MOH are the two serious consequences from the use of BCM.

A previous study described ten trials of BCM, but none was a well-done, randomized, controlled trial (RCT) [51]. A recent RCT was fairly negative for BCM [18]. The lack of RCTs for BCM reflects the era during which they were introduced. The paucity of trial evidence does not mean that BCM are not efficacious. We rely on anecdotal evidence for many of our older therapies. Although funding could be difficult, as these drugs are generic, it would be worthwhile to pursue at least one additional well-done RCT of BCM.

To minimize the risks of BCM, patient selection is crucial. I have found that the highest risk lies with those who have certain personality disorders, along with patients who previously overused addicting medications [80]. Patients with severe anxiety and/or depression may also be at risk for overuse. Reasonable limits on BCM might be: use restricted to 2 days per week and a limit of 20 tablets per month. There are outliers who do very well on 30–60 tablets of BCM per month, without MOH or addiction.

In an ideal world, BCM would not be necessary: preventive approaches would work well for a high percentage of patients, and our abortives would be headache specific, nonaddicting, and safe for all ages. We are a long way away from this ideal situation. If we eliminate BCM, many patients are left without effective options. We would not have BCM-mediated MOH, but many of these patients would subsequently overuse opioids, along with other analgesics. BCM have well-known downsides, but they also provide significant benefits. Note this letter originally appeared in *Headache,* Vol. 52, Sept. 2012.

## Medication Overuse Headache: Inaccurate and Overdiagnosed L. Robbins, M.D.

The article "Medication Overuse Headache" [53] is an excellent review. However, the entity "medication overuse headache" (MOH), as defined in the article, is misleading and inaccurate. Current diagnostic criteria for MOH only require abortive medication use on 10 or 15 days/month (depending upon the drug) [34]. What is not needed is any evidence that the abortive actually causes an increase in headache. Medication Overuse (MO) often occurs among people with frequent headaches. However, MO does not necessarily lead to increased headache. Diagnosing MOH is not an easy task. MOH diagnosis must require an individualized assessment of the patient's medication and headache history. The epidemiologic studies of MOH are not valid, as they do not differentiate MO from MOH.

A number of years ago all abortives, including nonsteroidal anti-inflammatory drugs (NSAIDs), were implicated in MOH. We now realize that certain drugs (NSAIDs and triptans) are less likely to cause MOH than others. Opioids and butalbital compounds are the worst offenders. Although simple NSAIDS usually do not contribute to MOH, they continue to be included in the MOH criteria.

Patients often are given the label of MOH simply because they admit to regularly consuming over-the-counter analgesics or a triptan. Many patients who frequently use these medications do not suffer from MOH. There are a number of variables, including genetics, age, type of drug, etc. that help to explain why one patient suffers from MOH, while the next does not.

For many patients with frequent headaches, behavioral techniques and preventive medications (including Botox) are inadequate. Our current preventives often provide little relief, and frequently cause unacceptable side effects. We do not have any preventives that were initially developed for headache. One long-term study indicated that only about half of migraineurs found any preventive helpful for longer than 6 months [65, 69]. Declining efficacy and increased side effects often lead to discontinuation of the preventive. Many physicians are quick to blame the patient for causing MOH. The patients are told that they are suffering from MOH due to a particular medication, even though: (1) they have only been taking that drug for a short time, (2) the headaches did not increase once they began the medication, or (3) drug withdrawal did not lead to a lessening of the headaches.

Physicians often instruct the patient to only use the abortive 2 days per week. The patient usually responds, "that is fine, but what do I do the other 5 days? I have to function." Many headache specialists and neurologists maintain a rigid posture, refusing to allow more than a bare minimum of abortive medication. The patient either suffers or drifts elsewhere.

Much of what is written about MO and MOH is confusing, with little basis in fact. These are arbitrary terms, without scientific validation. Of course, we must try to minimize abortives. Patients on frequent abortive medication should be withdrawn for a period of time, which is easier said than done. However, many refractory patients would have zero QOL without their (frequently used) abortives.

The current criteria conflate MO with MOH. As a result, MOH is wildly overdiagnosed. An inaccurate label of MOH may harm the patient. Patients with the MOH diagnosis often are denied the only medication that is helpful. We could redefine MOH, using scientifically validated criteria. Alternatively, we could drop the term MOH altogether. Note this letter originally appeared in the journal *Headache,* Nov/Dec, 2014.

## Difficult to Treat Headache: Patient Version

Refractory (difficult to treat headaches), which occur frequently, usually are CM. CM is defined as a headache occurring 15 (or more) days per month, of which at least 8 of the headaches are migraine. For those with CM, preventive medications often help. However, approximately one-half of patients with CM continue to suffer frequent pain, with little relief from medications. This condition is termed RCM.

RCM is described as frequent migraines that have failed adequate trials of various preventive and/or "as needed" medications. A person must have failed to obtain relief from at least two categories of preventive medications. In addition, the person with RCM usually has not found adequate help from the usual migraine "as needed" medications, such as sumatriptan, naproxen, etc. Those with RCM also find that their functioning and QOL is impaired by the frequent headaches. RCM affects millions of individuals.

A small minority of those with refractory headaches do not suffer from migraine. Instead, they may experience refractory cluster headaches or another headache syndrome.

Many questions involve RCM, such as:

What role does disability play, and should disability help define RCM?

How resistant to the myriad of available treatments qualifies the patient to be considered refractory?

Treatments may differ depending upon the age of the person; medications prescribed for a 16 year old may not be used at the age of 80. The resistance demonstrated by some patients may be due to genetics (genetics often plays a huge role), structural changes in the brain (particularly the white matter), and medication overuse.

Various subsets of RCM have been identified. These include posttraumatic headache, headaches exacerbated by medication overuse, headaches in a person with severe psychiatric illness, etc.

## *Outside of Medication*

The headache sufferer should not rely solely on medicine for relief. Lifestyle changes are important too. It is crucial to avoid caffeine overuse and to encourage "active coping," through exercise, physical therapy, yoga, psychotherapy, etc.

Exercise (at least, on average, 20 min daily) and weight control may improve headache and QOL. Yoga or Pilates may be beneficial. Physical therapy is often useful, and is primarily aimed at associated neck pain. Although stress may be a major trigger for the headaches, managing stress is difficult to achieve. For those with anxiety and/or depression, psychotherapy is helpful for improving QOL. Biofeedback and other relaxation techniques are also underutilized and should be considered.

Medication overuse headache (MOH) is a critical issue that must be addressed. It is important to try to limit "as needed" medications. If a patient is consuming pain medications or triptans for 10 or more days per month, he or she may be suffering from some degree of MOH. However, these analgesics often are the only effective treatment for that person. Withdrawal from the analgesics may be very difficult to accomplish. MOH tends to be overdiagnosed. Many patients overuse the pain or triptan medications. However, overuse of the "as needed" medicines does not necessarily mean that the drugs are increasing the headache.

## *Medication: Selected Outpatient Options*

When migraineurs have failed three or more of the "usual" preventive regimens (for example, topiramate, amitriptyline, beta blockers, etc), the physician should consider other treatment approaches. Most medications used for refractory headaches are considered "off-label:" they were initially developed for another purpose. How is a medication selected that is best suited for the individual? Comorbidities must be identified. These include the psychiatric and medical conditions, other than headaches, that occur in the individual. If someone has anxiety/depression, antidepressants may be prescribed. If weight gain is a major issue, drugs associated with weight gain must be avoided. With hypertension, medications used to lower the blood pressure are prescribed.

Each patient is unique, and our medication choices vary widely between patients. The following is a discussion of various treatment options for RCM.

## *Botulinum Toxin (Botox)*

Botulinum toxin type A (specifically Botox), is the only FDA-approved medication for CM. This treatment may be used once the diagnosis of CM has been established. Due to insurance or financial restrictions, Botox is usually injected after a number of other standard medications have failed. For CM, Botox is the most effective migraine preventive with the least side effects. Since 1996, over 3 million patients have received Botox for headaches. Botox is effective in 60–65 % of the patients, and the effects usually last for 2.5–3 months. Short-term side effects include eye drooping, headache, and neck pain. Long-term side effects have not been reported. The injections are minimally painful because Botox does not sting.

The FDA indication recommends Botox injections every 3 months. This totals 31 injections (155 units). Many patients do well with a lesser dose (60–100 units). Some physicians "chase the pain," injecting more Botox at the sites where the pain is located. If the Botox wears off after 2 months, it is generally safe to reinject before the 3-month interval.

Many insurance policies cover Botox injections, particularly with "prior authorization" obtained by the physician's office. An increasing number of physicians have received training in Botox injections for CM.

Most physicians, concurrently with Botox, also prescribe other preventive and "as needed" medications. For those patients with severe RCM, a multipronged approach is necessary, which includes nonmedication treatments, Botox, preventive agents, and "as needed" drugs.

## *Polypharmacy: Using Two (or More) Preventives*

Most patients with refractory headaches require more than one medication. Comorbidities "drive" the preventive approach. For example, topiramate which is an antiseizure drug approved for use in migraine prevention, is commonly used with the antihypertensive beta blocking agents (propranolol, timolol), which are also approved for migraine prevention. These drugs may be prescribed with other preventives, including the antidepressant amitriptyline. It is vital to minimize the drugs and to avoid side effects. For instance, if a person has constipation, we would avoid using the older antidepressants (such as amitriptyline). If weight gain is a problem, we may use topiramate instead of valproate. If a person cannot afford to have any memory problems (such as an accountant), topiramate may not be the best choice. For each migraineur, the "top ten" list of appropriate medications varies.

Concurrently with preventive therapy, almost all patients utilize "as needed" medications. The idea is to minimize the use of these drugs, trying not to "chase the headache" every 4 h. Most patients with RCM utilize one or two preventive agents, and three or four "as needed" drugs, from their medicine cabinet.

## *Daily (or Near-Daily) Triptans*

Some patients with migraine only respond to the triptans (sumatriptan, naratriptan, rizatriptan, etc.). Triptans have been available since 1991, and are relatively safe. Over the past 20+ years, several hundred million individuals have used triptans for their migraine attacks. Short-lasting side effects are often experienced, such as chest or neck pressure, tingling, fatigue, etc. Almost all patients who frequently utilize triptans (4 or more days per week), "self-select" this approach. Their physicians did not recommend daily use of triptan. The major issue with frequent triptan use is MOH. Although triptans may cause MOH, they are less likely to do so than analgesics containing caffeine, butalbital compounds, or opioids.

In addition to the risk of MOH, the major challenge of triptan use is cardiac effects. However, over the past 20 or more years, very few reports of cardiac problems have emerged. We are not certain of all the long-term risks of these drugs, but they may be safer than many alternatives. For example, one triptan per day is less harmful to the body than six aspirin with caffeine (or ibuprofen or naproxen) tablets. Many of the long-term side effects seen in headache patients are related to daily anti-inflammatory use. Most patients using triptans on a daily basis also have other "as needed" drugs to alternate with the triptan.

The ideal patient for triptan therapy experiences no triptan-related side effects and has minimal cardiac risk factors. Also, it is important to wean a patient from the triptan for a period of time, to ensure that MOH is not occurring due to triptan use. Cost and insurance reimbursements were previously a barrier to this approach. However, inexpensive generic triptans are now available.

## *Long-Acting Opioids (LAO)*

For a minority of RCM patients, LAO may provide the most effective relief. SAOs (Vicodin/Norco/Tylenol with codeine) only provide relief for 2–4 h, and have a high risk for MOH. The ideal LAO patient is one who has had excellent pain relief from SAOs, without overuse, and without tolerance to the analgesic effects. Tolerance occurs when a person requires constantly increasing doses in order to achieve the same effect. A person with a personality disorder (borderline, antisocial, narcissistic) is a poor candidate for LAO. Previous abuse of opioids or other addicting drugs increases the risk of MOH with LAO.

The use of opioids in patients under the age of 30 should be very restrictive. We rarely use LAO in younger patients. If a person has not used opioids on a daily basis, we are very hesitant to institute these drugs. It is important to avoid creating more headaches through the use of opioids. However, if an RCM sufferer has been using opioids for a prolonged time and fulfills the above criteria, they may respond well to an LAO. The "ideal" RCM patient for LAO would be: middle aged or older patient, the one who has tried many approaches, who no personality disorder, and has responded well to SAOs (good effectiveness with no overuse and no tolerance).

One key to using LAO is to minimize the dose; if high doses are required, the LAO will not be effective. Patients usually respond quickly to the LAO, enabling the physician to make an assessment after 4 weeks of treatment regarding effectiveness and side effects. If tolerance develops, whereby higher and higher doses are required, the LAO approach will not work for the long term.

A number of downsides to LAO have been identified, including: the risk for abuse or addiction, side effects such as fatigue or constipation, the stigma of taking daily opioids, difficulty obtaining the prescription, and dependence on the LAO (withdrawal may be difficult). However, for a small number of RCM patients, LAO greatly enhances their QOL. LAO may be safer over the long-term than the SAOs, because acetaminophen contained in the short-acting preparations may cause liver or kidney problems.

A number of LAO are available and usually do not contain acetaminophen, unlike the SAOs. Some patients respond well with buprenorphine (Butrans—a 7-day patch), while others prefer extended release morphine (Kadian—an excellent type of delivery system). Methadone has certain advantages (effective, can split tablets, inexpensive) and disadvantages (difficult withdrawal, more dangerous if overused). Oxycodone controlled-release (Oxycontin) carries a higher risk of abuse, and is much shorter acting than Butrans or Kadian. Zohydro is an excellent "pure" hydrocodone, without acetaminophen. Whichever type of LAO is used, it is crucial to only prescribe low doses.

## *Nerve Blocks*

Sphenopalatine ganglion (SPG) nerve blocks have been used for over 100 years. Several new devices are available that facilitate completing an SPG block in the physician's office. The SPG is a nerve center near the top of the nose, between the eyes. The block is accomplished easily, and takes only a minute. No pain has been reported. A type of novocaine is sprayed up the nose via the Tx360 or SphenoCath device. SPG blocks are safe, and most effective if done two or three times a week for several weeks. If effective, these blocks may provide relief for days or weeks (occasionally longer). Some neurologists and pain specialists perform the SPG blocks in their office.

Occipital nerve blocks involve injecting under the skin in the back of the head. Some type of novocaine is used, sometimes with cortisone. Although somewhat painful, occipital blocks are fairly safe. These injections may help for weeks (usually not more than one month). Some neurologists, and almost all pain specialists, perform occipital nerve blocks.

Trigger point injections are usually undertaken with a type of novocaine, injected into the neck or upper back areas. The effects of these injections may last from days to weeks, and are performed by some neurologists and pain specialists.

Deeper neck (cervical) injections may help some patients with RCM, particularly when the neck is involved. For those with neck and "back of the head" pain, these injections should be considered. These include steroid epidural injections, and "facet" nerve blocks which are performed by a pain specialist on an outpatient basis. Although generally safe, these injections carry slightly more risk than the superficial injections, and are costly.

## *Miscellaneous Medication Approaches*

Monoamine oxidase inhibitors (MAOI) are powerful antidepressants that may be effective for refractory headaches. For those with moderate or severe depression, the MAOIs may be beneficial.

Weight gain and insomnia are common side effects. With the traditional MAOI, such as phenelzine (Nardil), a low-tyramine diet must be followed, and certain medications may not be used concurrently. At this time, MAOIs, are probably underutilized. There is a milder MAOI patch available (selegiline, or Ensam) with less side effects.

Stimulants (methylphenidate or mixed amphetamine salts) may help pain as well as some comorbidities (fatigue, weight, attention). For some patients, these agents greatly enhance QOL. Fatigue is commonly encountered in headache patients, and stimulants may help offset the fatigue. Stimulants are primarily used for ADHD, which is a common condition. Many patients with RCM struggle with their weight, and the stimulants help in weight loss (at least for a period of time).

Methylergonovine (Methergine) is a medication used following childbirth, and is occasionally helpful for headaches. Methylergonovine is usually dosed 2 to 3 times daily. However, a number of medication interactions have been reported. Cost and availability have been issues.

Memantine (Namenda XR) is a drug used for memory problems (Alzheimer's syndrome). Memantine is fairly safe and well tolerated. Memantine (used in the XR form, once per day) is effective for some headache patients with very few drug interactions.

Muscle relaxants are occasionally effective for RCM. The nonaddicting agents are preferred, such as lioresal (Baclofen), cyclobenzaprine (Flexeril), or tizanidine (Zanaflex). Although generally safe, associated fatigue may limit their use. For those with insomnia, using a muscle relaxant at night may help both sleep and headache.

## *Conclusion*

For many chronic headache sufferers, the "usual" approaches are not effective. It is important to utilize nonmedication approaches while minimizing medicine. This article presents various treatment approaches for patients who have been unsuccessful with the standard headache therapies. Hopefully, in the near future, more effective therapies for pain will be available. It should be noted that most of the treatments discussed are not FDA approved for the indication of headache treatment. The therapies presented are this author's approach, and are not intended to represent "mainstream" treatment. This discussion is not prescriptive; the risks and benefits of any treatment should be discussed with your treating physician. Note that this article originally appeared in the patient journal Headwise; Vol. 4, Issue 2, 2014.

## Refractory Chronic Migraine: Long-Term Follow-up Using a Refractory Rating Scale

### *Introduction*

Refractory chronic migraine (RCM) is often a debilitating illness, with an enormous impact on QOL. The RHSIS of the AHS has provided a forum for physicians on this crucial topic. CM occurs in approximately 2% of the population [81]; the prevalence of RCM is unknown.

A lot of work has been accomplished on the definition of RCM [42]. A summary of the current proposed criteria are listed (see Table 2.11). The definition is a continuous work in progress [96]. Long-term outcomes for those with RCM have not been investigated. In addition, there is a range of severity among the RCM patients. For clinical and research purposes, it is important to categorize the RCM patients according to severity.

This study assessed pain and QOL in RCM patients over a 10 year period. A novel RCM "severity rating scale" was used for the evaluation of these patients.

**Table 2.11** Refractory chronic migraine criteria (Proposed) [96]

| |
|---|
| 1. Patient has diagnosis of chronic migraine (or migraine) |
| 2. Patient has failed adequate trial of at least two out of four drug classes |
| a. Anticonvulsants |
| b. Beta blockers |
| c. Tricyclics |
| d. Calcium channel blockers |
| 3. Patient has modified lifestyle and eliminated triggers |
| 4. Patient has failed abortive medications, including: |
| a. Triptans and DHE |
| b. NSAIDs and combination analgesics |
| 5. There may be modifiers: |
| a. With or without medication overuse |
| b. With significant disability |

*DHE* dihydroergotamine, *NSAID* nonsteroidal anti-inflammatory drug

# Methods

## Design and Patient Selection

This was a retrospective chart review of 129 RCM patients. RCM was diagnosed according to criteria suggested by the RHSIS of the AHS (Table 2.11).

**Inclusion Criteria** RCM patients older than 18 years as of the year 2000. The patients were followed at our headache center during the years 2000–2010, and must have remained at the clinic for that time. One hundred and twenty nine patients, with an average age of 49 (108 Females, ages 19–72 and 21 Males, ages 31–69), were assessed.

## Refractory Scale

A refractory scale of this author's design was utilized for assessment. The scale ranges from 2 (least severe) to 10 (most severe). See Table 2.12.

The patients were assigned a number (2–10) for severity as of the year 2000, and this assignment of severity was not reassessed after the initial date.

The severity groupings were as follows: score of 2, 3, or 4: mild RCM, score of 5, 6, 7: moderate RCM, score of 8, 9, 10: severe RCM.

**Table 2.12** Refractory scale (2–10, 10 = most severe)

| |
|---|
| 1. Refractory to preventives = 2 points (refractory to preventives is determined by RHSIS[a] and Silberstein [101] criteria) |
| 2. Refractory to abortives = 2 points (determined by RHSIS[a] and Silberstein[b] criteria) |
| 3. Greater than 10 years of chronic migraine = 1 point (chronic migraine defined according to International Headache Society (IHS) criteria [33]) |
| 4. Twenty five or more days of headache per month (on average) = 1 point |
| 5. Two of the following associated medical conditions: irritable bowel syndrome (IBS), fibromyalgia, temporal mandibular dysfunction (TMD), chronic pelvic pain, painful bladder syndrome, and chronic fatigue = 1 point. These syndromes were defined according to guidelines established by the various specialty organizations. Patients had to have been diagnosed using the standard criteria [47] |
| 6. Psychiatric comorbidities of the following types: severe Axis I (affective disorder), or any Axis II (personality disorder) = 1 point. These were diagnosed utilizing guidelines established in DSM-IV [3] |
| 7. Disability (work and/or home) = 1 point. Thepatient had to demonstrate moderate to severe disability with poor functioning for at least 6 months. Disability was assessed by various means, including interviews with the patient and family. A VAS functioning scale was utilized |
| 8. Medication overuse headache = 1 point. Criteria established by the IHS were utilized [33] |

*DSM-IV* Diagnostic and Statistical Manual of Mental Disorders, Fourth Edition, *RHSIS* Refractory Headache Special Interest Section *VAS* visual analog scale

## *Outcome Measures*

Quality of Life (QOL): QOL was measured by adding pain, functioning, and mood scores (each on a 1–10 scale, with 1 = best, 10 = worst). The QOL rating scale ranged from 3 (best) to 30 (worst). Pain was assessed via a visual analog scale (VAS) of 1–10, (10 = worst). Functioning was determined by the level of the work and/or home activities. Mood determinates included depression, anxiety, and insomnia. These were assessed using DSM-IV criteria.

Pain Level: Pain was assessed using a visual analog scale, 1–10 (10 = worst).

## *Statistics*

Statistical package for social sciences (SPSS) v17 for Windows was used for the statistical analyses. Difference scores for QOL1−QOL2 and pain ratings time1−time2 were calculated. In order to analyze if these pre-post scores differed across the three pain severity groups (mild, moderate, severe), a one-way analysis of variance (ANOVA) was conducted. To determine if the treatment was significantly effective in decreasing level of pain and improving QOL, pre-post paired samples *t*-tests were calculated for each severity group. Finally, Cohen's effect size formula [(mean1−mean2)/(the average of standard deviation1 + standard deviation2)] was used for paired samples *t*-tests.

# Results

$N = 129$ patients (108 F, ages 19–72, 21 M, ages 31–69, average age 49). The patients were initially categorized according to the refractory scale (2–10, 10 = most refractory). QOL (Table 2.13) and pain level (Table 2.14) were assessed as of the year 2000, and also as of the year 2010.

For the mild patients, 66 % improved by 30 % or more in QOL during these 10 years. In the moderate group, 57 % improved by 30 % or more, and in the severe group 61 % improved by 30 % or more.

QOL over 10 years was the same, or worse, in 4 % of mild patients, 16 % moderate, and in 18 % of severe patients.

ANOVA revealed significant mean change score (time1−time2) differences for QOL ratings between severity groups, $F(2126) = 4.31, p = 0.02$. Bonferroni post hoc results showed that improvements in QOL after treatment were significantly larger for the severe group compared to the mild group ($p = 0.045$) and for the severe group relative to the moderate group ($p = 0.03$). Change scores for the mild to moderate group did not significantly differ.

In the mild group, 80 % of the patients had a decline of 30 % or more in pain levels over the 10 years. In the moderate group, 72 % had a decline of 30 % or more

**Table 2.13** Quality of life: Year 2000 versus 2010

| Initial degree of refractoriness | Initial QOL in 2000 (3–30, 30 = worst) | Final QOL in 2010 | % Improvement in QOL, 2000–2010 |
|---|---|---|---|
| Mild (2–4 on refractory scale) $N=24$: average #=3.79 | 13.2 | 8.6 | 35% $p<0.001$, Effect Size(ES)=2.07 |
| Moderate(5–7) $N=67$: average #=6.04 | 15.8 | 10.8 | 32% $p<0.001$, ES=1.30 |
| Severe(8–10) $N=38$: average #=9.02 | 21.6 | 14.4 | 33% $p<0.001$, ES=1.50 |

**Table 2.14** Pain level: Year 2000 versus 2010

| Initial degree of refractoriness | Initial pain level (2000) (1–10, 10 = worst) | Final pain level (2010) | Change (%) from 2000–2010 |
|---|---|---|---|
| Mild (2–4) $N=24$ | 7.8 | 4.3 | −45% $P\cdot0.001$, Effect Size (ES)=2.55 |
| Moderate (5–7) $N=67$ | 7.7 | 4.5 | −42% $P\cdot0.001$, ES=1.30 |
| Severe (8–10) $N=38$ | 8.6 | 5.5 | −36% $P\cdot0.001$, ES=2.16 |

**Table 2.15** Overall results (Across all Groups) $N=129$

| | |
|---|---|
| Initial QOL(2000)=17 *(3–30 scale, 30=worst)* | Final QOL(2010)=11.4 *(33% improvement)* |
| Initial pain level(2000)=7.96 *(1–10 scale, 10=worst)* | Final pain level(2010)=4.76 *(40% improvement)* |

in pain levels. The severe group had 71% of patients reported a decline of 30% or more in pain over these 10 years.

Pain levels were the same, or worse, over the 10 years in only 4% of mild patients, 15% of moderate, and in 18% of the severe patients. ANOVA findings for the change scores in pain ratings failed to yield any correlation between severity group differences (Table 2.15).

Sixty percent of patients had an improvement in QOL by 30% or more (over the 10 years)

Fifteen percent of patients saw no change, or suffered a decrease, in QOL

Seventy three percent of patients had pain levels decrease by 30% or more

Fourteen percent of patients reported no improvement, or an increase, in pain levels over the 10 years

Paired samples *t*-tests were conducted for each severity group between assessment periods. In case of the mild group, QOL ratings significantly improved after treatment, $t(23)=11.88$, $p<0.001$, *ES* (Cohen's d)=2.07, and pain ratings significantly decreased, $t(23)=10.15$, $p<0.001$, $ES=2.55$.

**Table 2.16** Medications. The following medications were reported to be beneficial by the refractory patients. To be listed, the patient must have found the medication helpful for their pain, and to have continued on the medication for at least 6 months

| | Opioid | Frequent triptans, 4+ per week | Butalbital | Onabotulinum-toxinA | Stimulant | Other |
|---|---|---|---|---|---|---|
| Mild<br>*N*=24 | 10<br>42 % | 11<br>46 % | 3<br>13 % | 6<br>25 % | 4<br>17 % | 2<br>8 % |
| Moderate<br>*N*=67 | 44<br>66 % | 23<br>34 % | 11<br>16 % | 9<br>13 % | 5<br>7 % | 6<br>9 % |
| Severe<br>*N*=38 | 27<br>71 % | 6<br>16 % | 8<br>21 % | 6<br>16 % | 6<br>16 % | 4<br>11 % |
| Total<br>*N*=129 | 81<br>63 % | 40<br>31 % | 22<br>17 % | 21<br>16 % | 15<br>12 % | 12<br>9 % |

In the moderate group, QOL significantly increased, $t(66)=9.95$, $p<0.001$, $ES=1.30$, and pain levels significantly decreased, $t(66)=13.36, p<0.001, ES=2.26$. Finally, results for the severe group revealed a statistically significant increase in QOL after treatment, $t(37)=9.51, p<0.001, ES=1.50$, and a significant decrease in pain levels, $t(37)=10.42, p<0.001, ES=2.16$. Overall, the results suggested that the treatment was effective in improving QOL, and reducing level of pain for all severity groups (Table 2.16).

Overall, the medications that helped the most over the 10 years included: opioids (63 %), frequent triptans (31 %), butalbital compounds (17 %), and onabotulinumtoxinA (16 %).

## Discussion

This study categorized RCM patients according to a unique refractory rating scale. The patients were evaluated as of the year 2000, and again 10 years later. Most (60 %) of the patients had at least a 30 % improvement in QOL, while 73 % also experienced a 30 % (or more) improvement in pain levels. While the severe patients also improved over 10 years, they still had significantly lower QOL, and higher pain scores than the mild or moderate patients. In this refractory group, opioids and frequent triptans were the most commonly used medications.

The refractory rating scale presented here is an initial attempt to classify RCM patients according to severity. A refractory scale may be beneficial for both clinical and study purposes. Patients with mild RCM will generally be easier to treat than those with severe RCM. Therapeutic studies on those with RCM may be less likely to succeed if the patients have severe RCM versus milder RCM. The individual components of the scale reflect various elements of refractoriness, including comorbidities. This author awarded more weight to “refractory to preventives” (2 points) or “refractory to abortives” (2 points) than to the other components (1 point each), primarily because refractory to preventives or abortives are central hallmarks of RCM.

As the plasticity of the brain may be an important factor in refractoriness, it is important to include the length of time of the headache (selected for this study at > 10 years). The average number of headache days per month is important, with 25 + days probably being more refractory than 15–24. Associated medical comorbidities often occurring in those with CM were included. These conditions may complicate treatment, and add to refractoriness. For this study, we included the following: IBS, fibromyalgia, TMD, chronic pelvic pain, painful bladder syndrome, and chronic fatigue.

Psychiatric comorbidities, commonly seen in RCM patients, certainly complicate treatment. Significant abuse in childhood may predispose one to RCM. Important comorbidities include anxiety, depression, the bipolar spectrum, personality disorders, somatization, and posttraumatic stress disorder [75, 78]. For this study, severe DSM-IV Axis I (affective disorders), or any Axis II (personality disorders) were considered important in refractoriness [3].

Disability should be a part of a refractory scale. Those who function at a low level, at work or at home, often are more resistant to treatment. Patients exhibit a wide range of coping and resilience. Resilience is a combination of nature and nurture; one can almost predict resilience based upon the shape of the serotonin transporter gene. This author believes that disability, or a chronically low level of functioning, renders it less likely that the RCM will improve. The level of functioning should factor into a refractory rating scale.

Medication overuse headache (MOH) is a remarkably complicated concept; MOH must be distinguished from medication overuse without resulting headache. It can be exceedingly difficult to determine who has MOH [33]. For this study, we used IHS guidelines as to MOH. MOH does add to refractoriness and resistance to treatment, and should be included in a refractory scale [33].

The medications utilized by patients in this study included: opioids (usually LAO), frequent triptans, butalbital, onabotulinumtoxinA, and stimulants. The author has published on most of these subjects [71, 72, 77, 79]. For RCM patients, it often takes a combination of medications to achieve even minimal benefits. Many of the patients in the study took two or more of the listed medications.

RCM constitutes a small but important subset of migraine patients. For clinical and study purposes, it is helpful to categorize RCM patients as to the degree of refractoriness. After 10 years, the severe patients remained behind the other groups regarding QOL and level of pain. However, over the 10 years, all of the groups (mild, moderate, severe) improved regarding QOL and level of pain. This initial attempt to create a refractory rating scale should be refined and improved with further study and research. Note this article originally appeared in The Journal of Headache and Pain, Vol. 13, 2012.

## Comment Observation and Rebuttal

### *Long-Acting Opioids and Headache*

The article by Morris Levin, MD, "Opioids in Headache," [43] is an excellent review of the subject. I agree that LAO may be beneficial for a small number of refractory patients with CM. In addition, those with severe, refractory posttraumatic headache, as well as new-onset daily persistent headache may be good candidates. Over time I have developed guidelines for patient selection for LAO, which include:

1. The patient must truly be refractory to multiple other approaches.
2. We should not use these medications under the age of 30, with rare exceptions.
3. Exclude certain personality disorders, particularly borderline, antisocial, and paranoid. (I have not found anxiety, depression, or bipolar to be a substantial risk factor for LAO.)
4. There must have been a good response to shortacting opioids, without escalation of dose and lacking significant side effects.
5. Patients should be excluded if they previously overused/abused short-acting opioids.
6. Use low doses; if patients need escalation they are probably not good candidates.
7. Heed red flags, particularly early in treatment; early problems with abusive behaviors rarely lead to successful long-term treatment.

My long-term success with LAO improved from 22% during the 1990s to 42% from 2000 to 2008, and is now 48% (currently 46 patients total) [70, 76]. This primarily reflects a 20-year learning curve as to patient selection. In addition to improved selection, we now have more choices of LAO (particularly the buprenorphine patch).

Dr. Levin discusses MOH from opioids; while MOH is certainly a major problem, the patients selected for LAO should have successfully been taking short-acting opioids, without increased headache. Dr. Levin also raises the possibility of OIH; OIH is certainly encountered, but not everyone develops OIH, and these candidates must have had a significant decrease in head pain from opioids, not an increase.

Dr. Levin states that "tolerance to the analgesic, euphoric and relaxing effects seems to be inevitable for most patients taking opioids chronically." This is true, but for those who do not develop analgesic tolerance, the LAO may be a good choice. I have treated a number of patients who have remained on the same low opioid doses for up to 20 years. In virtually all of the successfully treated LAO patients, tolerance to the euphoric effects wanes over time.

The patients who are candidates for LAO tend to be in the "severe" RCM group [82]. QOL is abysmal for these people. The treatment choices (polypharmacy, intravenous treatments, MAO inhibitors, stimulants, nerve stimulation, nerve blocks, etc.) often are ineffective or are poorly tolerated. Certainly LAO is only appropriate for a small minority of refractory patients, and often is not successful for a long term [92, 93]. In a number of years, we will have significantly improved treatments for these patients. Until then, we should consider LAO for the occasional refractory patient who fits our guidelines.

Lawrence Robbins, MD
Robbins Headache Clinic, Northbrook, IL, USA

## Suggested Readings

1. Akiskal HS, Bourgeois ML, Angst J et al (2000) Re-evaluating the prevalence of and diagnostic composition within the broad clinical spectrum of bipolar disorders. J Affect Disord 59(Suppl 1):S5–S30
2. American Pain Society (2002). Guidelines for the management of pain in osteoarthritis, rheumatoid arthritis and juvenile chronic arthritis, 2nd edn. American Pain Society, Glenview
3. American Psychiatric Association (1994) Diagnostic and statistical manual of mental disorders, 4th edn. American Psychiatric Association, Washington DC
4. American Psychiatric Association (2000) Diagnostic and statistical manual of mental disorders, 4th edn. (Revised; DSM-IV-TR). American Psychiatric Association, Washington DC
5. Ashkenazi A, Silberstein S (2008) Botulinum toxin type A for the treatment of headache: why we say yes. Arch Neurol 65(1):146–149
6. Atluri S, Sudarshan G (2002) A screening tool to determine the risk of prescription opioid abuse among patients with chronic nonmalignant pain. Pain Physician 5(4):447–448
7. Biederman J, Wilens T, Mick E, Spencer T, Faraone SV (1999) Pharmacotherapy of attention-deficit hyperactivity disorder reduces risk for substance abuse disorder. Pediatrics 104(2):e20
8. Butler SF, Budman SH, Fernandez K, Jamison RN (2004) Validation of a screener and opioid assessment measure for patients with chronic pain. Pain 112(1–2):65–75
9. Butler SF, Fernandez K, Benoit C, Budman SH, Jamison RN (2008) Validation of the revised screener and opioid assessment for patients with pain (SOAPP-R). Pain 9(4):360–372
10. Casavant M (2002) Urine drug screening in adolescents. Pediatr Clin North Am 49(2):317–327
11. Chabal C, Erjavec MK, Jacobson L, Mariano A, Chaney E (1997) Prescription opiate abuse in chronic pain patients: clinical criteria, incidence and predictors. Clin J Pain 13(2):150–155
12. Chen F, Fishman S, Kreis P (2008) The opioid contract. In: Smith HS, Passik SD (eds) Pain and chemical dependency. Oxford University Press, New York, pp 359–365
13. Cicero TD (2007) The development of a comprehensive risk management program for prescription opioid analgesics. Pain Med 8:157–170
14. Conway S, Delplanche C, Crowder J, Rothrock J (2005) Botox therapy for refractory chronic migraine. Headache 45(4):355–357
15. Dahlof CG, Mathew NT (1998) Cardiovascular safety of 5HT1B/1D agonists—is there cause for concern? Cephalagia 18:539–545
16. Dahlof CG, Falk L, Risenfors M, Lewis C (1998) Safety trial with the 5HT1B/1D agonist avitriptan (BMS-180048) in patients with migraine who have experienced pressure, tightness, and/or pain in the chest, neck, and/or throat following sumatriptan. Cephalalgia 18:546–551
17. Dalal S, Melzack R (1998) Potentation of opioid analgesia by psychostimulant drugs: a review. J Pain Symptom Manage 16:245–253
18. DeRosier F, Sheftell F, Silberstein S et al (2012) Sumatriptan- naproxen and butalbital, a double-blind, placebo-controlled crossover. Headache 52:672–674
19. Diamond S (1993) Tension-type headaches. In: Dalessio DJ, Silberstein SD (eds) Wolff's headache and other head pain, 6th edn. Oxford University Press, New York, p 249

20. Doleys DM, Cornelius D, Watters S, Marino M (2008) Long-term therapy using short acting opioids for chronic non-cancer pain. Pract Pain Manage 8(4):40–50
21. Drago F, Caccomo G, Continella G, Scapagnini U (1984) Amphetamine-induced analgesia does not involve brain opioids. Eur J Pharmacol 101:267–269
22. Dunbar SA, Katz NP (1996) Chronic opioid therapy for nonmalignant pain in patients with a history of substance abuse: report of 20 cases. J Pain Symptom Manage 11(3):163–171
23. Farrar JT, Young JP Jr, LaMoreaux L et al (2001) Clinical importance of changes in chronic pain intensity measured on an 11 point numerical pain rating scale. Pain 94:149–158
24. Finkel R, Cubeddy LX, Clark MA (2008) CNS stimulants. In: Harvey RA, Champe PC, Finkel R, Cubeddy LX, Clark MA (eds) Lippincott's illustrated reviews: pharmacology, 4th edn. Lippincott Williams and Wilkins, Philadelphia, pp 117–127
25. Fishman SB (1999) The opioid contract in the management of chronic pain. J Pain Symptom Manage 18(1):27–37
26. Food and Drug Administration (2014) FDA allows marketing of first device to relieve migraine headache pain. http://www.fda.gov/newsevents/newsroom/pressannouncements/ucm378608.htm. Accessed 18 Aug 2014
27. Gallagher R (2004) Opioids in chronic pain management: navigating the clinical and regulatory challenges. J Fam Pract 53(10 suppl):s23–s32
28. Goadsby PJ, Hargreaves R (2008) Refractory migraine and chronic migraine: pathophysiological mechanisms. Headache 48(6):799–804
29. Gokani T, Robbins L (2002) Botulinum toxin: efficacy in migraine, tension-type and cluster headache. Am J Pain Manage 12:98–103
30. Gourlay D, Heit H (2008) Urine drug testing in pain and addiction medicine. In: Smith HS, Passik SD (eds) Pain and chemical dependency. Oxford University Press, New York, pp 353–357
31. Guyuron B, Reed D, Kriegler JS, Davis J, Pashmini N, Amini S (2009) A placebo-controlled surgical trial of the treatment of migraine headaches. Plast Reconstr Surg 124:461–468
32. Haas DC, Sheehe PR (2004) Dextroamphetamine pilot crossover trials and n of 1 trials in patients with chronic tension-type and migraine headache. Headache 44(10):1029–1037
33. Headache Classification Committee of the International Headache Society (2004) The international classification of headache disorders, 2nd edn. Cephalagia 24(suppl 1):1–160
34. Headache Classification Committee of the International Headache Society (IHS) (2013) The international classification of headache disorders, 3rd edn. Cephalalgia 33(9):629–808
35. Hillis WS, Macintrye PD (1993) Sumatriptan and chest pain [letter, comment]. Lancet 342:683
36. Inturrisi C (2008) Opioid pharmacology for pain. In: Smith HS, Passik SD (eds) Pain and chemical dependency. Oxford University Press, New York, pp 175–182, 189
37. Jaffe LA (1987) The prediction of drug use among college students from MMPI, MCMI and sensation-seeking scales. J Pers Assess 51(2):243–253
38. Kalso E, Edwards JE, Moore RA, McQuay HJ (2004) Opioids in chronic non-cancer pain: a systemic review of efficacy and safety. Pain 112:372–380
39. Katz NP, Adams EH, Chilcoat H et al (2007) Challenges in the development of prescription opioid abuse-deterrent formulations. Clin J Pain 23:648–660
40. Krishnan KR (2007) Revisiting monoamine oxidase inhibitors. J Clin Psychiatry 68(suppl 8):35–41
41. Laux G, Volz HP, Moller HJ (1995) Newer and older monoamine oxidase inhibitors: a comparative profile. CNS Drugs 3(suppl 2):145–158
42. Levin M (2008) Refractory headache: classification and nomenclature. Headache 48(6):783–790
43. Levin M (2014) Opioids in headache. Headache 54:12–21
44. Lipton RB, Bigal ME (2008) Toward an epidemiology of refractory migraine: current knowledge and issues for further research. Headache 48(6):791–798
45. Lipton RB, Bigal ME, Diamond M et al (2007) Migraine prevalence, disease burden, and the need for preventive therapy. Neurology 68(5):343–349

46. Lloyd K (1994) The clinical profile of sumatriptan: safety and tolerability. Eur Neurol 34(Suppl 2):40–43
47. Longo D, Fauci A (2011) Harrison's principles of internal medicine: vol 1 and 2, 18th edn. McGraw Hill Professional, New York
48. Mao JP (1995) Mechanisms of hyperalgesia and morphine tolerance. Pain 62:259–274
49. Mathew P (2013) A critical evaluation of migraine trigger site deactivation surgery. Headache doi:10.1111/head.12218
50. Mathew NT, Kurman R, Perez F (1990) Drug induced refractory headache—clinical features and manage- ment. Headache 30:634–638
51. McCrory DC, Goslin RE, Gray RN (1998) Evidence report: butalbital-containing compounds for the treatment of tension-type and migraine headache. Duke University Center for Health Policy Research, Raleigh
52. Mellick GA, Mellick LB (1998) Cluster headache management with methylphenidate (Ritalin). Headache 38(9):710–712
53. Munksgaard SB, Jensen RH (2014) Medication overuse headache. Headache 54(1):1251–1257. doi:10.1111/head.12408
54. National Institute of Mental Health (2014) Mania symptoms and bipolar disorder II more likely to lead to substance abuse than depression. http://www.nimh.nih.gov/news/science-news/2008/mood-disorders-predict-later-substance-abuse-problems.shtml. Accessed 25 Aug 2014
55. Oshinsky ML (2004) Botulinum toxins and migraine: how does it work? Pract Neurol 2004(suppl):10–13
56. Passik S, Kirsh K (2008) Chemical coping. In: Smith HS, Passik SD (eds) Pain and chemical dependency. Oxford University Press, New York, pp 300–301
57. Portenoy RK (1996) Opioid therapy for chronic nonmalignant pain: a review of the critical issues. J Pain Symptom Manage 11:203–217
58. Dodick D, Turkel C et al (2010) OnabotulinumA for treatment of chronic migrain: Preempt clinical program. Headache 50(6):921–936
59. Raja SN, Haythornwaite JA, Pappagallo M et al (2002) Opioids versus antidepressants in post-herpetic neuralgia: a randomized placebo-controlled trial. Neurology 59:1015–1021
60. Rapaport MH (2007) Dietary restrictions and drug interactions with monoamine oxidase inhibitors: the state of the art. J Clin Psychiatry 68(suppl 8):42–46
61. Rapoport AM, Bigal ME, Volcy M, Sheftell FD, Feleppa M, Tepper SJ (2003) Naratriptan in the preventive treatment of refractory chronic migraine: a review of 27 cases. Headache 43:482–489
62. Richman JA, Shinsako SA, Rospenda KM et al (2002) Workplace harassment/abuse and alcohol related outcomes: the mediating role of psychological distress. J Stud Alcohol 63(14):412–419
63. Robbins L (1996) Daily opioids (methadone) for refractory chronic daily headache. Headache Q 7(1):39–42
64. Robbins L (1997) Long-acting opioids (methadone) for refractory chronic headache: quality of life assessment. Headache Q 8(3):234–236
65. Robbins L (1999a) Long-acting opioids for severe chronic daily headache. Headache Q 10(3):135–139
66. Robbins L (1999b) Oxycodone CR, a long-acting opioid for severe chronic daily headache. Headache Q 10(4):305–308
67. Robbins L (2000a) Management of headache and headache medications, 2nd edn. Springer-Verlag, New York, pp 58–64
68. Robbins L (2000b) Tension headache preventive medication. In: Robbins L (ed) Management of headache and headache medications, 2nd edn. Springer, New York, pp 109–113
69. Robbins L (2001) We need better preventives (Letter). Headache 41:611–612
70. Robbins L (2001) Long-acting opioids for chronic daily headache. Pain Clin 3:13–15
71. Robbins L (2002) Botulinum toxin: efficacy in migraine, tension-type and cluster headache. Am J Pain Manage 12:98–103

72. Robbins L (2004) Frequent triptan use: observations on safety issues. Headache 44:1–5
73. Robbins L (2004) Frequent triptan use: observations on safety issues. Headache 44(2):172–182
74. Robbins L (2007) The bipolar spectrum in migraine, cluster and chronic tension headache patients. US Neurol Dis 3(2):30–31
75. Robbins L (2008) The bipolar spectrum in migraine, cluster and chronic tension headache. Eur Neurol Rev 3(1):123–124
76. Robbins L (2009) Long-acting opioids for refractory chronic migraine. Pract Pain Manage 9(6):45–54
77. Robbins L (2009) Long-acting opioids for refractory chronic migraine. Pract Pain Manage 9(6):74–78
78. Robbins L (2009) The prevalence of Personality disorders in migraineurs. Pract Pain Manage 9(1):52–54
79. Robbins L, Maides J (2009) Efficacy of stimulants in migraneurs with comorbidities. Pract Pain Manage 9(7):58–59
80. Robbins L (2010) A practice guide for continuous opioid therapy for refractory daily headache (Letter). Headache 50:1614
81. Robbins L (2010) Refractory chronic migraine. Pract Pain Manage 10:10–24
82. Robbins L (2012) Refractory chronic migraine: long-term follow-up using a refractory rating scale. J Headache Pain 13:225–229
83. Robbins L, Maides J (1999) Efficacy of preventive medications for chronic daily headache. Am J Pain Manage 9(4):130–133
84. Robbins L, Maides J (2000) Long-term daily triptan use: 59 patients. Headache Q 11(4):275–277
85. Robbins L, Goldfein P (2008) Personality disorders and the bipolar spectrum. Pract Pain Manage 8(3):46–50
86. Robbins L, Maides J (2009) Efficacy of stimulants in migraineurs with comorbidities. Pract Pain Manage 9(7):58–59
87. Rothrock J (2005) Methadone therapy in refractory chronic migraine. Headache 45(6):830
88. Rothrock J (2008) Treatment-refractory migraine: the case for opioid therapy. Headache 48(6):850–854
89. Rothrock JD (2005) Methadone therapy in refractory chronic migraine. Headache 45(6):830
90. Rothrock JF (2008) Treatment-refractory migraine; the case for opioid therapy. Headache 48(6):850–854
91. Saper JR, Lake AE 3rd (2008) Continuous opioid therapy (COT) is rarely advisable for refractory chronic daily headache: limited efficacy, risks and proposed guidelines. Headache 48(6):838–849
92. Saper JR, Lake AE, Bain PA et al (2004) Daily scheduled opioids for intractable head pain: long-term observations of a treatment program. Neurology 62:1687–1694
93. Saper JR, Lake AE, Bain PA et al (2010) A practice guide for continuous opioid therapy for refractory daily headache: patient selection, physician requirements, and treatment monitoring. Headache 50:1175–1193
95. Savage S (2002) Assessment for addiction in pain-treatment settings. Clin J Pain 18(4 suppl):s28–s38
95. Schulman EA, Lake AE III, Peterlin B et al (2007) Defining refractory migraine and chronic migraines: proposed criteria from the refractory headache special interest section (RHSIS) of AHS: OR15. Headache 47:747
96. Schulman EA, Lake AE III, Goadsby PJ, Peterlin B et al (2008) Defining refractory migraine and refractory chronic migraine: proposed criteria from the Refractory Headache Special Interest Section of the American Headache Society. Headache 48:778–782
97. Schulte-Mattler WJ, Leinisch E (2008) Evidence based medicine on the use of botulinum toxin for headache disorders. J Neural Transm 115(4):647–651
98. Sheftell FD, Rapoport AM, Coddon DR (1999) Nara- triptan in the prophylaxis of transformed migraine. Headache 39:506–510

99. Silberstein SD, Lipton SR, Solomon S, Mathew NT (1994) Classification of daily and near daily headaches: pro- posed revisions to the IHS classification. Headache 34:17
100. Silberstein S, Lipton R, Dodick D (2007) Wolff's headache and other head pain, 8th edn. Oxford University Press, New York, p 159
101. Silberstein S, Dodick D, Pearlman S (2010) Defining the pharmacologically intractable headache for clinical trials and clinical practice. Headache 50:1499–1506
102. Smith HS, Vanderah TW, McCleane G (2008) Opioids for pain. In: Smith HS, Passik SD (eds) Pain and chemical dependency. Oxford University Press, New York, pp 183–202
103. Smith T (2001) Cardiovascular and safety concerns in using triptans in migraine patients. Headache Q 12(suppl 1):25–28
104. Stricker BH, Ottervanger JP (1992) Chest pain due to sumatriptan (see comments). Ned Tijdschr Geneeskd 136:1774–1776
105. Tfelt-Hansen PC, Diener H-C (2012) Why should American head-ache and migraine patients still be treated with butalbital- containing medicine? Headache 52:530–543
106. Vandevenne MV (2000) Detection time of drugs of abuse in urine. Acta Clinica Belgica 55(6):323–333
107. Visser WH, de Vriend RH, Jaspers MW, Ferrari MD (1996) Sumatriptan in clinical practice: a 2-year review of 453 migraine patients. Neurology 47:46–51
108. Watson CP, Watt-Watson JH, Chipman ML (2004) Chronic non-cancer pain and the long term utility of opioids. Pain Res Manage 9:19–24
109. Webster LW (2005) Predicting aberrant behaviors in opioid-treated patients: preliminary validation of the opioid risk tool. Pain Med 6(6):432–442
110. Webster LR, Dove B (2007) Avoiding opioid abuse while managing pain. Sunrise River Press, North Branch, pp 48–89
111. Zeppetella GR (2006) Opioids for the management of breakthrough (episodic) pain in cancer patients. Cochrane Database Syst Rev 1:CD004311

# Chapter 3
# Child and Adolescent Headaches

## Child and Adolescent Headaches

A multidisciplinary approach—a balance of medication with therapy and lifestyle changes—is the most helpful for children with severe headaches to help them return to normal functioning in home, school, and social life.

Headache is a common complaint among children and adolescents. The prevalence of migraine in those with headache varies by age and gender throughout childhood and adolescence. Migraine begins earlier in boys than in girls and, until the age of 7, migraine occurs slightly more often among boys. By menarche, the prevalence of migraine in boys and girls is roughly equal. However, after menarche, migraine begins to predominate among females and this gender separation increases even further in late adolescence.

Headaches, especially migraines, have a significant impact on the lives of young people. Approximately 65–80 % of children with migraine headaches will experience disruption of their normal daily activities at home, in school, and other social settings. The burden of migraine may also result in the development or worsening of anxiety or depression. Because of the quality of life issues, early recognition and management of headaches in children and adolescents is crucial.

Headache disorders can be categorized as either primary or secondary. As with adults, the vast majority of headaches in children and adolescents are primary headache disorders: migraine (with or without aura), tension-type headache, and chronic daily headache.

Secondary headache disorders, although much less common, may be due to various organic etiologies which can range from the relatively benign to the serious. Such underlying organic conditions include:

- Bacterial causes: acute febrile illness, rhinosinusitis, dental abscess, intracranial and extracranial infections;
- Systemic illness: hypertension, diabetic ketoacidosis;
- Miscellaneous: head or neck trauma, vascular malformations, subarachnoid hemorrhage, intracranial mass lesions, etc.



L. Robbins, *Advanced Headache Therapy*, DOI 10.1007/978-3-319-13899-2_3

## *Diagnostic Approach*

Although headache can be a presenting symptom of underlying organic pathology, accurate information from the patient and family is often enough to identify or rule out the most serious etiologies. The overwhelming majority of headache disorders are diagnosed by a thorough history and physical examination. A complete medical and psychiatric history, family history, medication history (including prescription, over-the-counter, and vitamins/herbs), allergy history, and social history should also be obtained.

Migraine tends to be underdiagnosed; patients and their parents often attribute headaches and nausea to "the flu" or dismiss them as "sinus headaches." Careful attention must be paid to the patient's description of headache onset, timing, frequency, duration, severity, quality, location, precipitating factors, and aggravating or alleviating factors. Associated symptoms—especially nausea, vomiting, photophobia, and phonophobia—are often the key to an accurate diagnosis of migraine.

Potential indicators of organic pathology can include severe vomiting, a headache which awakens a child from sleep, and the absence of a family history of migraine. Also, progressive, unremitting daily pain, neurologic symptoms, and fevers are important. If any of these red flags are present, the appropriate laboratory and imaging investigations should be performed.

In a patient with an unremarkable history, where a primary headache disorder is suspected, laboratory investigation is usually not warranted beyond baseline laboratories. These usually include, but are not limited to, a complete blood count and metabolic panel.

Neuroimaging studies are usually not indicated in children with a normal neurologic examination and a history consistent with a primary headache disorder, especially migraine or tension-type headache. These children will not usually have significantly abnormal findings on head computed tomography (CT) scans or intracranial magnetic resonance imaging (MRI). A small percentage may have incidental and/or unrelated findings, but routine neuroimaging is not absolutely indicated in children with typical primary headaches.

MRI is the preferred test of the brain; usually it does not need to be done with contrast. MRI is important for those with new onset headaches, atypical head pain, or abnormal neuro symptoms or signs.

Usually, electroencephalography (EEG) is not helpful in the routine diagnostic assessment of pediatric headache patients. However, an EEG should be performed on patients with an atypical migraine aura, episodic loss of consciousness, or symptoms suggestive of a seizure disorder. Background slowing may be seen during some migraine attacks, but the EEG results are usually normal.

Lumbar puncture (LP) is indicated if meningitis, encephalitis, subarachnoid hemorrhage, or high–low pressure syndromes are suspected. Cerebrospinal fluid and pressure measurement should also be performed. In those patients where increased intracranial pressure is suspected—or in those with focal neurologic deficits—a head CT scan or similar neurologic imaging modality should be performed prior to an LP . We attempt to avoid the LP unless absolutely indicated. However, if meningitis or encephalitis is suspected in a toxic-appearing patient, treatment should not be delayed in order to perform the head CT scan first.

## *Biopsychosocial Approach*

For those with more severe or frequent headaches, a comprehensive biopsychosocial approach is needed. This approach requires the collaboration of medical and behavioral specialists working together to improve a patient's overall functioning and the quality of life. The combination of both pharmacologic and nonpharmacologic treatments is ideal for those with frequent headaches. Nonpharmacologic treatments are particularly important as they are typically more effective in children and help to minimize medications and side effects.

## *Nonpharmacologic Treatments*

Nonpharmacologic modalities consist of patient education, lifestyle strategies, behavioral interventions, physical therapy, etc. Patient education should be the first step taken. Legitimizing the headache as a physiological disorder is of primary importance. It helps to say "…Migraines are a genetic medical condition, like asthma or diabetes…"

Children and their parents usually want to hear three things from the physician: (1) the cause of the headache (including triggers), (2) the treatment and prognosis, and (3) reassurance that a primary headache disorder is not serious. It is important that realistic goals and expectations are set. Children and their parents should understand that there are no miracle cures for headaches.

It is usually helpful to introduce the use of a headache diary as a means to identify specific triggers. Of course, some triggers (e.g., weather changes, stress, hormonal influences) cannot be avoided, but certainly many—such as missing meals, bright lights/sunlight, undersleeping/ oversleeping, foods, perfume, cigarette smoke, and certain types of physical exertion—can be managed. Headache diaries should record the frequency and severity of headaches as well as document the efficacy and side effects of treatments. Using a diary will improve the patient's or parents' recall of the headaches and make office visits more productive. They can also help persuade children and adolescents of the need for lifestyle changes.

Lifestyle strategies should include an emphasis on proper diet, exercise, and sleep habits. Headache patients do better with regular schedules, eating three or more meals per day, and going to bed and awakening at the same time every day, including weekends. Daily exercise can be particularly helpful; patients should strive for at least 30 min of exercise per day. Generally, headache patients do better with low-impact exercises such as swimming, walking, biking, and yoga.

Behavioral interventions—such as psychotherapy, counseling, and relaxation techniques—may be helpful for many adolescents who experience significant stress in their lives. Overscheduling adds to the usual adolescent stressors. The incidence of hard-driving perfectionistic behavior and depression is increased in adolescents with severe headache. Children and adolescents who miss substantial blocks of time in school or social activities need to be assessed for depression, school phobia, and secondary gains. Counseling for children, as well as family-centered therapy for children and their parents, is often helpful in promoting active coping and is an indispensable augmentation to medical therapy.

Relaxation techniques such as biofeedback, deep breathing, and imaging should be encouraged. Most adolescents can learn relaxation techniques from books or audiovisual aids that are readily available. However, seeing a therapist who teaches biofeedback is much more effective. Most children under the age of 10 cannot learn and apply biofeedback, but some as young as seven can learn simple breathing and imaging techniques.

## *Pharmacologic Treatment*

There are two types of pharmacologic treatments for headaches: abortive and preventive. Decisions on medication depend upon the frequency and severity of the headaches and how much they bother the patient. Some children are not overly bothered by their daily headaches and tend to ignore them. Others may be incapacitated and miss an entire year of school.

As with adult headaches, abortive medication is used in the overwhelming majority of cases without daily preventive medication. Patients should be encouraged to use their abortive medication early, while their headaches are mild. Early intervention is a key step in successful use of migraine abortives. See Table 3.1 for a list of first-line abortive medications.

It is always reasonable to try biofeedback together with simple abortive medications as the first step and attempt to avoid daily preventive medication, if possible. However, with frequent migraines, or for moderate to severe daily headaches, daily preventive medication may be necessary. In order to minimize medications, start at a low dose of a daily preventive and slowly titrate up to reasonable efficacy. Table 3.2 has a more complete list of criteria for the use of preventive medication. Table 3.3 lists first-line preventive medications.

Realistic goals and expectations for medications need to be discussed. For abortive medications, the goal is to achieve significant relief (>70%) as quickly as possible. When preventive medications are used, the goal is to reduce headache frequency and severity by 30% or more and to improve functioning. Patients may note that the efficacy of their abortive medications improves with the use of a daily preventive.

When preventive medications are used in children and adolescents, it is prudent to periodically attempt to discontinue the daily preventive in an effort to minimize medications. In choosing a preventive, comorbidities (anxiety, depression, gastrointestinal (GI) problems, etc.) "drive" where we go with which medication. As with adults, the idea is to see if the patient may return to simply using abortive medication. However, if an adolescent has had headaches for a number of years and has found a preventive that works, the usual practice is to continue it long term.

**Table 3.1** First line abortive medications for migraine and tension-type headaches in children and adolescents

| *Under 12 years of age* |
|---|
| 1. Ibuprofen: Effective, and available as a liquid, but GI upset is relatively common. A small amount of caffeine may enhance the efficacy |
| 2. Acetaminophen: Well tolerated, safe, but not as effective as ibuprofen. Chewable tablets and liquid are available. Due to its relative safety, acetaminophen is the usual primary abortive used in young children. Adding a small amount of caffeine may enhance efficacy |
| 3. Naproxen (Naprosyn, Aleve): Effective abortive that is nonsedating and is available as a liquid. However, GI side effects are common. (Aleve=OTC=220 mg) |
| 4. Midrin (generic available) or Prodrin: Midrin capsules: (acetaminophen 325 mg/dichloralphenazone 100 mg/isometheptene 65 mg): ½ or 1 capsule PO q 4 h prn. At younger ages we usually use only ½ at a time. These are very large capsules, but may be taken apart and sprinkled into applesauce or juice. Sedation is common, as is lightheadedness. GI upset, although not common, occurs at times |
| Prodrin is very similar to Midrin, but without the sedative (no dichloralphenazone), and with a small amount (20 mg) of caffeine. Prodrin tablets may be split in half |
| 5. Caffeine: Used by either itself or with an analgesic, caffeine is useful for tension and migraine headache. In children, soft drinks containing caffeine are helpful. Side effects are minimal when caffeine is used in very limited amounts |
| 6. Triptans: Rizatriptan (Maxalt) is indicated for age 6 and above. Maxalt is available in 5 and 10 mg, in tabs or MLT lozenges. The usual dose would be 5 mg, ½ to start, and increasing dose with advancing age. There is a very low dose sumatriptan nasal spray available (5 mg). I usually begin using the triptans at age 9 or 10 |
| 7. (Last resort) Butalbital or other pain medications: Phrenilin (generic available) is butalbital plus acetaminophen, while Fioricet/Esgic adds in caffeine. These should be used in low doses(usually ½ tablet) and not more than 1 day per week |
| *Over 12 years of age (includes the above plus the following)* |
| 8. Triptans: Almotriptan (Axert tablets) is FDA-indicated in adolescents. We usually begin with ½ tablet. Maxalt is FDA-indicated age 6 and above. Zomig nasal spray is available in a low dose, 2.5 mg, form (the usual dose in adults is 5 mg). Triptans are generally more effective than analgesics. Contraindicated in complicated migraine and in those with cardiovascular risk factors. Potential side effects include flushing, chest tightness, paresthesias, nausea, and somnolence. More effective when taken early. May be combined with NSAIDs (ibuprofen, naproxen) |
| 9. Prodrin: Acetaminophen, isometheptene, caffeine. Similar to Midrin, but nonsedating. These may be cut in ½, and taken with an NSAID |
| 10. NSAIDs or Cambia: Most NSAIDs may be used with or without caffeine. Cambia is FDA-indicated above age 18, but has been used off-label in adolescents. Cambia is 50 mg, in powdered form, of diclofenac potassium. Cambia may be used with water or apple juice, and the usual dose is ½ or 1 packet every 4 h as needed |
| 11. (Last resort) Butalbital or other pain medications. See above |

*GI* gastrointestinal, *OTC* over the counter, *FDA* Food and Drug Administration, *NSAID* nonsteroidal anti-inflammatory drug

**Table 3.2** Criteria for the use of prevention medication

| |
|---|
| 1. The headaches interfere significantly with the child's functioning socially or at school. The extent of how much the headaches bother the child is a major consideration |
| 2. Failure of nonpharmacological approaches (watching triggers, biofeedback, etc.) |
| 3. The child's and parent's willingness to utilize daily medication with possible side effects |
| 4. Willingness of the child and parents to change medication, if necessary |
| 5. Failure of abortive medication to effectively treat the headaches; continued frequency of headaches, daily or near-daily |
| 6. In choosing preventives, comorbidities (psychiatric, medical, GI) drive where we go |

*GI* gastrointestinal

**Table 3.3** First-line preventive medications for migraine, tension-type, and chronic daily headaches in children and adolescents

| |
|---|
| *Under 12 years of age* |
| 1. Cyproheptadine: Safe, but efficacy is questionable. It is usually well tolerated but fatigue and weight gain may be a problem. Not as useful in children over the age of 11. It may be dosed once a day and is available in liquid form |
| 2. NSAIDs (Ibuprofen, naproxen): Ibuprofen and naproxen may be utilized as daily preventives or as abortive for both tension and migraine headaches. The lack of sedation renders these very helpful for daily use. GI side effects are relatively common, and when these are used on a long-term basis, regular blood tests for hepatic enzymes and renal function need to be done |
| 3. Petadolex. (Age 9+): A form of the herb butterbur. Good evidence for efficacy in migraine. Widely used in Europe; available for over 35 years and regarded as safe. One tablet (50 mg) daily; may increase to two. Occasional mild GI upset. May be ordered through www.petadolex.com, 1-888-301-1084, or through Amazon.com. Due to carcinogenic concerns (in animal studies, although Petadolex takes off the molecule that is of concern, from the parent compound butterbur), we recommend rotating off of Petadolex for at least 1 month periodically |
| 4. Magnesium oxide or citrate: Available OTC as tablets or powder. Mild, but effective for some. Safe in this age range. Usual dose is 100–200 mg a day |
| 5. Feverfew (natural, herbal) is sometimes effective |
| 6. Topiramate or divalproex: see below: we attempt to avoid these drugs in younger children, but occasionally they are utilized, in low doses |
| 7. Botox: Off-label under age 18. Botox is the most effective chronic migraine preventive; occasionally Botox has been used under age 12, in low doses |
| *12 years and older* |
| 1. NSAIDs: occasionally effective for prevention, without the sedative/weight gain side effects of many drugs |
| 2. Petadolex: See above. Magnesium also is used at all ages |
| 3. Topiramate: Useful for both migraine and chronic daily headache (CDH), lower doses (e.g., 25–50 mg qHS) are often effective; may be pushed to 100–150 mg daily. Potential side effects include cognitive slowing, paresthesias, decreased appetite/weight loss, and rarely acute glaucoma, renal stones, and acidosis. Cognitive side effects often limit use |
| 4. Divalproex: Useful for both migraine and CDH, lower doses (e.g., 250 mg) are usually used with some efficacy. May be pushed to 750–1000 mg daily. Potential side effects include GI upset, sedation, weight gain, tremor, dizziness, and alopecia. Blood tests should be performed periodically for hepatic enzymes |

**Table 3.3** (continued)

| |
|---|
| 5. Gabapentin: Useful for both migraine and CDH, lower doses (e.g., 100–300 mg BID to TID) are often effective. Potential side effects include dizziness and weight gain, although it is usually very well tolerated by most people, especially at the lower doses recommended |
| 6. Tricyclic antidepressants: Effective for migraine and CDH. Nortriptyline and amitriptyline are commonly used. Usually well tolerated in low doses and safe for long-term use. Cognitive side effects, dry mouth, drowsiness, dizziness, and weight gain are common. Usual dose of amitriptyline is 10–50 mg daily. Protriptyline does not cause weight gain, but is somewhat less effective. Blood tests should be performed periodically for hepatic enzymes and renal function |
| 7. Propranolol: Generally well tolerated. Fatigue and decreased exercise tolerance may be a problem. Usual dose is 20–80 mg daily. With doses less than 60 mg qd, BID dosing is required which is inconvenient for children |
| 8. Verapamil: A calcium channel blocker that is effective for migraine and occasionally CDH. Generally well tolerated, with constipation common. Convenient once per day dosing with the sustained release formulations. Usual dose ranges from 80 mg once a day up to 240 mg ER q day |
| 9. Botox: Off-label under age 18; botox is only officially indicated for chronic migraine, 18 and above. Botox has been studied in this age range, and is generally regarded as safe and effective. Despite being off-label, Botox has been widely utilized in the 12–18-year age range. The official (age 18 and above) doses are 155 units, given as 31 injections about the head. For younger patients we often use much lower doses, with fewer injections |

NSAID nonsteroidal anti-inflammatory drug, GI gastrointestinal, OTC over the counter

## *Conclusion*

Many children and adolescents have episodic migraines that respond easily to abortive medications. The challenge is in dealing with those who have frequent and debilitating headaches. A multidisciplinary approach is the most helpful for patients with severe headaches: a balance of medication with therapy and lifestyle changes. Management of headache disorders is a trial and error process; there is no "cookie cutter" approach. Although decreasing the frequency and severity of headaches is important, success is also measured by how much we help the child return to normal functioning in home, school, and social life. Note this is an updated version of an article that was originally in *Practical Pain Management*, Vol. 10, Jan. 2010.

## The Homebound Adolescent Headache Patient

Each adolescent with refractory headaches is unique, and requires an individualized approach. This involves the parents, siblings, school, and health-care villagers (physicians and therapists) working together with the goal to decrease pain and increase function.

I have an adolescent headache center north of Chicago. Years ago, I would take a simplistic, tough love approach: "…My job is to come to work; yours is to go to school, no excuses." I have evolved toward a more nuanced approach, individualized to each child's situation.

In the case of chronic refractory headache patients, we are not simply treating one child in isolation; we are also dealing with the parents, siblings, and the school. Long-term outcomes with these children somewhat depend upon the psychiatric health of the parent. The primary "caretaker" parent (usually the mother) can range from psychiatrically normal to those with a severe personality disorder (PD). The child's psychiatric status is also a crucial variable. It "takes a village" to raise some of these children, and we recruit "other villagers." These include psychotherapists, physical therapists, biofeedback specialists, etc.

## *Role of Therapist Is Key*

Adolescent psychotherapists are invaluable in treating these patients. They often provide the most useful treatment for the child. Many therapists will take a family therapy approach. Family dynamics play a crucial role in perpetuating refractory headaches. Also, the patient's severe headaches adversely affect the rest of the family. Many of the kids are not ready for high school, and have tremendous fears and anxieties. After a number of sessions, the therapist often has a good grasp on why the child has severe headaches, along with school avoidance. For some kids, the long-term relationship with the psychotherapist may be the most important element of treatment.

## *Mental Health of Parent Is Important*

The psychiatric health of the parent (usually mom) is also important. The most difficult case is when the mother has a PD, most often borderline PD (BPD), and the child has a PD. Except in severe cases, we reserve diagnosing an adolescent as having a PD until their later teens or early 20s. With plasticity of the brain, children diagnosed with BPD may significantly improve by age 25 or 30. I have followed a number of patients into their 20s, and when both mother and child are psychiatrically ill, the result is not good. These patients often underfunction as young adults, never leaving home or finishing school.

When mom has a BPD, she may perpetuate a mild factitious disorder by proxy (FDP; Munchausen by proxy). I published an article on this situation, where we evolved into taking a dialectical approach with both mom and adolescent [7]. Dialectical therapy is used with BPD, and with these mothers I call it "dialectical by proxy." Basically, this means we are nonconfrontational, "go with the flow," trying to minimize medical interventions, and maximize psychotherapy. Confronting the BPD parent leads to an angry scene, with the parent (and child in tow) stomping out of the office, never to be seen again. With the milder approach, I have had several children actually separate from the mother after high school, and do reasonably well. Separation is vital if the child is to mature into a relatively healthy adult.

## *Ease into a School Program*

Many children need a tough love approach and must be pushed to go to school. Others do best with home schooling or when homebound, online education, modified school (limited hours in class), or a hybrid. Homeschooled kids may do reasonably well academically, but they risk ending up being socially isolated. Homebound-schooled adolescents often experience severe anxiety, and not attending school may help alleviate their social anxiety. Each child's needs differ. Not all schools are flexible, and alternative programs may not be available.

When a homebound child returns to school, it is helpful to ease back into school. I will usually write letters recommending late starts, early release, no gym, etc.—whatever helps. If the adolescent is at least willing to go back to school part-time, I will do my part and help facilitate the return to school. This works for some of the children.

The idea is to go from point A (Ninth grade) to point B (graduating high school). Some children accomplish this by taking the general educational development (GED) exam. It may take part homeschooling, part regular high school, going for two classes in summer—whatever works. If we can help these children progress through high school, and separate them from mom, they usually function better into their late teens and 20s.

## *Somatizing Disorders*

Many children with refractory headaches are somatizers—that is, patients with frequent physical complaints for which no organic basis is found. They tend to visit multiple physicians and other providers. I minimize testing with these patients, and almost never hospitalize them. It is important to move away from the medications and medical establishment, and help these children see themselves as healthy, not chronically ill.

As with adults, active coping (taking responsibility for one's illness) is key. Pain level itself is not the only predictor of disability in these children. Other predictors include catastrophizing (thinking illness is worse than it actually is), fear of pain, passive (vs. active) coping, depression, and anxiety [3–5]. We can work on "dialing down the volume" on catastrophizing, both in the child and parent. I see "catastrophizing by proxy," where a parent may say: "These headaches are the worst anybody has ever had. They are a 12 on a scale of 1–10. It is a nightmare. You have to cure them!" Encouraging active coping is a major challenge. We need to have the parent, teacher, therapist, etc., on the same page. If the parent (and child) state: "When you give enough drugs to stop the pain, then he will go back to school," that never works out well.

### *Summary*

My approach to the refractory headache patient has evolved over the years toward a flexible case-by-case approach. I encourage active coping and always minimize use of medications. I attempt to work with other health-care providers ("villagers"), particularly psychotherapists. One goal, outside of helping to decrease the pain, is to gently facilitate a separation of adolescent from parent. Each adolescent with refractory headaches is unique, and requires an individualized approach. Note this is an updated version of an article that originally appeared in *Practical Pain Management*, Vol. 13, April 2013.

## Factitious Disorder in an Adolescent with Headaches

### *A Case of Mild Factitious Disorder by Proxy*

**History** Jason is a 14-year-old boy who presents with multiple pain disorders, dating to age 7. Medical history includes previous diagnoses of chronic Lyme disease, chronic migraine, fibromyalgia, chronic fatigue syndrome, and irritable bowel syndrome. Jason missed most of eighth grade this past year, but has done well with homebound education. Oddly, Jason's records do not corroborate his stated diagnoses.

Jason's mother (Ellen) and father accompany him to his first visit, and Ellen does almost all of the talking. His father is very quiet and defers to his wife. Jason has one older sibling, who still lives in the home while commuting to college.

Ellen appears very excited when telling us about Jason's various medications, doctors, and tests. Jason is on two antidepressants "for pain," an anticonvulsant, nonsteroidal anti-inflammatory drugs (NSAIDs), and muscle relaxants. He has physicians in three states, and averages two doctor visits a week.

On the surface, Ellen is very friendly and courteous. She tells us about an upcoming sleep study in which Jason will be participating, as she is convinced her son has a sleep disorder, "…but the doctors missed it on the first sleep study." Overall, she is very dissatisfied with his medical care. When we suggest that Jason see a psychotherapist, or have psychological testing, Ellen agrees, stating he will go, "as soon as he is finished with all his other tests."

### *Introduction*

There are a number of warning signs in this case that point to a factitious disorder: multiple diagnoses lacking solid medical evidence; multiple patient visits to a number of physicians in various locations; repeated medical tests; and a caretaker requesting more tests, doctors, and diagnoses. The mother's demeanor and affect are typical of parents in the mild FDP situation: very friendly, overly interested, excited and involved, and dissatisfied with the medical care.

The caretakers, usually the mother, often have PDs themselves, with narcissistic tendencies. If they are confronted, anger and splitting can ensue. Confrontation and honesty may work with healthy parents, but not with very psychiatrically ill parents.

Our goal is to gently nudge Jason and his family toward psychotherapy, and to minimize medications and tests. We want to ensure Jason is able to go from freshman year of high school through his senior year. We eventually want to separate Jason from his mother with his departure for college. It takes a unified effort to help a child and family in this situation, and we must recruit others, particularly mental health professionals.

## Diagnosis

This case represents mild FDP, as well as pediatric condition falsification (PCF) [1, 2, 6, 8–10].

## Treatment

There are two treatment approaches that can be considered.

**Approach 1** We establish a therapeutic relationship, and determine that Jason is not being poisoned or seriously harmed, other than psychologically, by the mother. Then, at a later date, we confront Jason's parents with our true thoughts.

**Approach 2** We pursue a low key, nonconfrontational approach to both the parents and children. Dialectical therapy, using acceptance, mindfulness, validation, and cognitive-behavioral techniques, among other tools, is currently our favored approach. After years of failure following confrontations with parents, I have used this laid-back "dialectical by proxy" approach with two young patients and their mothers, with reasonable success. One young woman currently is doing well in college, having physically separated from her parents. If our goal is to continue a therapeutic relationship, and ease the young person away from home, I believe that this approach may be best.

## Long-Term Follow-Up

Over the 25 years I have been in practice, I have seen ten patients with mild FDP/PCF. Five patients have been lost to follow up (usually after we confronted the parent). Two patients have done well into their 20s, and are not considered to have

PDs. One young woman was diagnosed with BPD, and has done poorly. Another young woman is doing well in college, and a 15-year-old has improved, and is attending high school part-time. My impression is that, after the vitally important separation from parents, many victims may do well as adults, as long as they themselves do not have a PD.

## *Discussion*

The sample case represents a mild form of FDP, mild PCF, and possibly mild medical child abuse (MCA). FDP is primarily a psychiatric diagnosis that relates to the caregiver who exaggerates or completely fabricates the child's symptomatology. PCF relates more to the child/victim, who has had symptoms falsified. MCA relates to the health-care providers, who may prescribe unnecessary and possibly harmful treatments, including drugs. The MCA diagnosis recognizes the role of health-care providers in the abuse of the child.

The incidence of FDP is not entirely known, but is relatively rare. The incidence has been quoted as ranging from 0.4 to 2 cases per 100,000 (among parents of children younger than 16 years of age). Boys and girls appear to be equally affected, and, typically, younger children are involved. However, with mild FDP presenting as headaches, we have witnessed most cases occurring in early adolescence. The incidence of the milder forms of these conditions is unknown.

## *The Participants*

The three participants are the child/victim, the parent/perpetrator, and the health-care team. The child (or adolescent) often is passive, deferring to the caretaker, who, regardless of the age of the patient, does almost all of the talking. Older children may collude with the parent. The adolescent often is dependent and immature, with separation anxiety.

The perpetrator parent, 90 % of whom are the mothers, often is very attentive, knowledgeable, overly friendly, and comfortable in the medical setting. The vast majority of these parents have moderate to severe psychopathology, often some form of PD. Some of the mothers display hypochondriacal traits, and occasionally have been involved in factitious disorders themselves. The caretakers that we have encountered with mild FDP are essentially "doctor addicts," and are not actively inducing physical symptoms in the children. They seek various types of secondary gain, including sympathy, attention, and social interaction with the medical staff, and relief from their usual chores or work, and so on.

The role of the Internet has grown over the years. Parents can obtain a great deal of medical knowledge without being part of a health-care environment. Many of the perpetrators display a wealth of knowledge about the various conditions, although it tends to be superficial. Also, angry parents may use the Internet to post negative statements about health-care providers.

The health-care team is the third participant. Often, the primary provider is a subspecialist, eager to help with an unusual diagnosis. Health-care providers have widely different levels of psychiatric acumen, and often ignore or miss obvious signs of FDP. In moderate or severe cases, it is more obvious as to the correct course, with psychiatric intervention, as well as legal notification of Child Protective Services. However, with mild cases, the correct means of intervention are not as clear.

## *Treatment*

Management of these conditions varies from case to case. It "takes a village" to help these families, and we need other "villagers." These often include psychotherapists, psychiatrists, social workers, the pediatrician, and so on. With moderate and severe cases, legal intervention is important. However, with the milder cases that I have seen over the years, the correct course is unclear. In the majority of the first seven cases I encountered, confrontation usually led to an angry scene, with the parent stalking out of the office, never to return. In three more recent situations, I have taken a more subtle "dialectical" approach, which has been much more successful. One case was that of a 15-year-old girl with severe daily headaches and multiple diagnoses; she was not in school for 2 years. We gently guided her into individual and family therapy, with little confrontation, and she is now off to college and doing well. Most of the time, however, the parents will resist or refuse psychotherapy. It is apparent that the correct approach to mild FDP/PCF is not known, and we need research and studies on this milder form. Note this is an updated version of an article that was published in *Practical Pain Management*, Vol. 11, Oct. 2011.

## Suggested Reading

1. Criddle L (2010) Monsters in the closet: Munchausen syndrome by proxy. Crit Care Nurse 30(6):46–55
2. Fujiwara T, Okuyama M, Kasahara M, Nakamura A (2008) Differences of Munchausen syndrome by proxy according to predominant symptoms in Japan. Pediatr Int 50:537–540
3. Kashikar-Zuck S, Vaught MH, Goldschneider KR, Graham TB, Miller JC (2002) Depression, coping, and functional disability in juvenile primary fibromyalgia syndrome. J Pain 3(5):412–419
4. Martin AL, McGrath PA, Brown SC, Katz J (2007) Anxiety sensitivity, fear of pain and pain-related disability in children and adolescents with chronic pain. Pain Res Manag 12(4):267–272
5. Milde-Busch A, Boneberger A, Heinrich S et al (2010) Higher prevalence of psychopathological symptoms in adolescents with headache: a population-based cross-sectional study. Headache 50(5):738–748
6. Pankratz L (2006) Persistent problems with Munchausen by proxy label. J Am Acad Psychiatry Law 34(1):90–95
7. Robbins L, Bassett B (2011) Teenage boy with multiple pain disorders. Pract Pain Manage 11(8):12–14

8. Shaw RJ, Sayal S, Hartman JK, DeMaso DR (2008) Factitious disorder by proxy: pediatric condition falsification. Harv Rev Psychiatry 16(4):215–224
9. Squires JE, Squires Rh Jr. et al (2010) Munchausen syndrome by proxy: ongoing clinical challenges. J Pediatr Gastroenrol Nutr 51(3):248–253
10. Stutts JT, Hickey SE, Kasdan ML (2003) Malingering by proxy: a form of pediatric condition falsification. J Dev Behav Pediatr 24(4):276–278

# Chapter 4
# Cluster Headache

## Cluster Headache

*Summary of cluster headache characteristics and update on abortive and preventive treatments*

Cluster headache is among the most severe pains known to mankind. It is characterized by excruciating, debilitating pain lasting from 15 to 180 min, or occasionally longer. The pain is usually located around or through one eye or on the temple. The series of cluster headaches usually lasts several weeks to several months, once or twice per year. Clusters may occur every other year, or even less frequently. Several of the following are usually present: lacrimation, nasal congestion, rhinorrhea, conjunctival injection, ptosis, miosis of the pupil, or forehead and facial sweating. Nausea, bradycardia, and general perspiration also occur in many patients. Attacks usually recur on the same side of the head. Cluster headaches tend to occur more in spring and fall. There is usually no family history of cluster headache, but occasionally there is such a family history.

### *Specific Characteristics of Cluster Headaches*

Males are afflicted more than females by a 2.5:1 ratio. The onset of the clusters is usually between the age of 20 and 45, but there are many cases of clusters in teenagers and occasionally clusters begin in the 50s or 60s and rarely in the 70s. Women tend to have an older age of onset for their cluster headaches than men. Occasionally, a brief aura may occur. The prevalence is 0.4 % of the population. See Table 4.1 for a summary of characteristics.

The pain of the cluster attack is extreme and starts very quickly, usually without an aura or a warning. Within minutes, it becomes very severe. Although the pain is usually located about the eye or temple, it may be more intense in the neck or facial areas. Although usually unilateral, the pain changes sides in 10–15 % of patients—



L. Robbins, *Advanced Headache Therapy,* DOI 10.1007/978-3-319-13899-2_4

**Table 4.1** Typical characteristics of patients with cluster headaches

| |
|---|
| Begins between ages 20 and 45, approximately 0.4% of the population |
| Male predominance in a 2.5 : 1 ratios |
| Same time of year with no headache in between the cluster cycles |
| Primarily nocturnal attacks (but may be anytime) |
| During cluster cycle, alcohol triggers the headaches |
| Severe, excruciating, unilateral pain—usually periorbital |
| Ipsilateral rhinorrhea, lacrimation, conjunctival hyperemia, sweating of the forehead, Homer's syndrome |

either during a cluster cycle or the next cycle may see pain on the opposite side. The pain itself is excruciating, described in various manners as sharp, stabbing—"like my eye is being pulled out" and occasionally, throbbing.

The length of attack varies, but 45 min is the average. Cluster patients usually experience one or two headaches per day, but this may increase to as many as seven per 24 h or decrease to as little as one or two per week. They usually occur around the same time each day, with the time period 9 p.m. to 10 a.m. being the most frequent. Approximately, half of the patients awaken from sleep with the headaches.

Cluster cycles, except in the chronic variety, usually last 3–8 weeks and then stop until the next bout of clusters. The clusters occasionally last as little as several days, or as long as 5 months at which time we begin to think that they may have converted to the chronic cluster type. Ten percent of cluster patients have chronic clusters in which there is no break of at least 6 months between attacks. One or two bouts of the clusters per year are average for most patients. They may increase in frequency with only several months in between bouts or several years may elapse between attacks. When periodic clusters begin at older ages, the chance of conversion to chronic cluster becomes greater. The natural history of clusters is not known, but the tendency is for the cluster series to stop at a certain age. Many patients "lose" their clusters in the late 30s or 40s, particularly if they have had them for many years.

During the cluster series, over half of the patients are very sensitive to alcohol and most patients will have an attack triggered by ingestion of alcohol. The other "headache foods" are less important, but avoiding monosodium glutamate (MSG), aged cheeses and meats, and chocolate is prudent during the cluster series. MSG, in particular, seems to trigger a more sever cluster in some patients. Cluster patients may have their clusters after stress is over and occasionally excessive cold, heat, or bright light have been associated with the precipitation of a cluster. However, most cluster patients have very little control over the clusters, except with medication.

The typical episodic cluster series builds over 1–2 weeks and peaks for 1–3 weeks and then decreases. In the 10% of cluster patients with chronic clusters, periods of peaks and valleys with the headaches also occur but an extended break without any clusters is not present. Chronic clusters are not usually consistent throughout the year but tend to increase in certain seasons. In managing the clusters, we keep in mind the fact that the clusters build and then peak so that I often treat them with somewhat less medication—particularly corticosteroids—in the beginning of a cluster period. The natural history of clusters is unknown. However, it appears as if the more years a patient has them, the more likely they are to abate.

## Nonmedication Treatment of Cluster Headache

Other than medication, very little is available for sufferers of cluster headache. The pain is too severe for relaxation methods and some patients state that biofeedback or relaxation may actually precipitate or increase a cluster. However, learning simple deep breathing techniques or relaxation methods does aid some patients in helping to curb the anticipation of the cluster attacks. Much anxiety is generated during the day when the patient knows that nighttime brings intense, excruciating pain.

Icing the area of pain may help, although sometimes heat will be more effective. Some patients let the shower run hot water on their cervical area, or they use a shower water massage apparatus to allow the hot water to run over their cervical or frontal area. Pressing over the temporal area with moderate pressure is occasionally helpful. Cluster patients usually feel better when moving about during an attack. They tend to be active (such as pacing) as opposed to the quiet sought by migraineurs.

## Medications for Cluster Headache

For most patients, both abortive and preventive medications are helpful and only in a minority of situations do we simply use abortive medicines.

The abortive treatment for clusters is the same for episodic and chronic cluster headaches. Since the headache is very intense from the beginning and the pain is severe and excruciating, medication to aid the attack must act quickly. Most cluster attacks last less than 1 h, averaging about 45 min, and thus oral pain medication is only of limited value. However, in patients whose attacks do last for more than 1 h, pain medications may be useful—particularly if the standard cluster abortives are not completely effective. Antiemetics are also used for those patients with nausea, and the sedative effect of these is often helpful.

## First-Line Cluster Abortive Medications

The first-line cluster abortive medications are as follows:

- Inhaled oxygen
- Sumatriptan injections
- Imitrex® (sumatriptan) or Zomig® (zolmitriptan) nasal spray

**Oxygen** Oxygen is effective in approximately 70 % of cluster headache patients. To obtain a small tank with a mask is relatively easy and not terribly expensive. The tanks are usually rented for 1 month. If feasible, most patients with cluster headaches should attempt to use oxygen for their attacks. The patient should be sitting with the body leaning slightly forward. A mask is used and 100 % oxygen is inhaled at 12–15 L/min. In healthy patients with no pulmonary problems, the oxygen may be inhaled for 15–20 min. A rebreather mask is helpful.

**Sumatriptan Injections** Injectable sumatriptan (Imitrex®, Sumavel™, or generic: prefilled syringes, vials, EpiPen of sumatriptan, Stat Dose System) is generally effective. Sumatriptan pills are more helpful for migraine than for cluster headache, but oral triptans are occasionally adequate. Many patients are reluctant to give themselves injections but, for those who are willing, injected sumatriptan is usually effective—often within minutes—and with a minimum of side effects. Oxygen may be used in conjunction with sumatriptan, and escape pain medication may also be utilized.

The dosage of sumatriptan is usually 4–6 mg given subcutaneously at the onset of the cluster headache. A repeat dose may be given at least 1 h after the first injection. Two injections, or 12 mg, is the maximum recommended dosage per 24 h. Sumatriptan is administered subcutaneously by the use of a convenient auto-injector device. Sumavel™ DosePro™ is a "needle-free" sumatriptan injection. While Sumavel is convenient, it still does sting, and may bruise quite a bit. Also, vials of sumatriptan are available for use with an insulin syringe. By using the vials, the dose may be titrated (some cluster patients only require 3 or 4 mg).

Daily use of sumatriptan has not been studied extensively. Thus, until further studies are known, prudent use of sumatriptan would dictate that no more than six injections per week be taken for cluster headache (less for migraineurs).

The side effects of sumatriptan are generally less than those with dihydroergotamine (DHE). Transient pain at the site of injection is common, and "icing" the injection site prior to use may decrease this burning pain. Other side effects include tingling sensations, disturbances of taste, heat flashers, and feelings of pressure or heaviness. Side effects tend to be short lasting. Chest symptoms, flushing, dizziness, and overall weakness may also occur. Minor transient increases in blood pressure have been seen. Nausea is relatively common. Sumatriptan should not be used in children, in pregnant women, in the presence of hepatic or renal impairment, or with cardiovascular disease. Patients over the age of 45 should be screened for cardiac risk factors. The frequent chest pressure that occurs is not usually felt to be of cardiac origin.

Sumatriptan or (Zomig) zolmitriptan nasal spray: while not as effective as the injection for cluster headache, the nasal spray is very convenient and many patients prefer this route of administration. We usually limit the sprays to two per day, but for cluster headaches we will occasionally utilize a third spray as well. Of the two nasal sprays, Zomig nasal spray 5 mg is more effective than the sumatriptan spray. There is a 2.5-mg Zomig nasal spray available, but the vast majority use the 5-mg spray. While not as rapidly effective as the injections, the nasal spray works faster than triptan tablets. Speed is essential in relieving cluster headache, yet occasionally patients prefer the oral triptans.

## *Second-Line Cluster Abortive Medications*

Second-line therapies include oral triptans, ergots and DHE, Cambia, ketorolac nasal spray or injections, oral pain medications, and intranasal lidocaine.

**Oral Triptans** Any of the oral triptans may help, but are usually too slow for cluster headache. Sumatriptan 100 mg is the most commonly used oral triptan. The two slow-acting triptans, frovatriptan and naratriptan, are not usually used acutely for clusters. Occasionally, these longer-acting triptans are utilized, mostly at night, to prevent nocturnal clusters.

**Ergotamine Tartrate** Strong vasoconstrictors, the ergotamines, have many limitations. Ease of administration (they are available as tablets) is a major advantage of the ergots. The frequent side effects of nausea and nervousness limit their use. In older patients, the risk of angina or an actual myocardial infarction restricts its use. The rebound headaches that occur in migraineurs do not seem to be as prevalent a problem in cluster headache patients. The primary ergotamine preparations are generic Cafergot® pills, suppositories and Ergomar® sublingual pills. Peripheral vascular disease or hypertension (HTN) is a contraindication. Ergotamines may exacerbate peptic ulcer disease. The effective dose of ergotamine varies widely among patients. Ergots may be combined with the use of oxygen and other abortive measures but not with triptans.

**Ergomar** Tablets contain 2 mg of ergotamine tartrate with no caffeine. The usual dose is one pill sublingually at the onset of the cluster attack. Ergomar may also be swallowed and this route may be just as effective as the sublingual method. This may be repeated once in 1 or more hours and limited to two pills per 24 h. Nausea is a common side effect as is a bitter or "bad" taste in the mouth. Nervousness is a frequent side effect, but less so than with Cafergot because there is no caffeine in Ergomar. Ergotamines need to be used with great caution in the presence of HTN, peripheral vascular disease, or peptic ulcer disease. If chest symptoms occur, ergots should be discontinued.

**Generic Cafergot (only generic available)** Consists of 1 mg of ergotamine tartrate and 100 mg of caffeine. Cafergot pills are the most convenient but least effective of the ergots. Dosage is one or two pills at the onset of headache, repeated every 2 h as needed, with a maximum of four per day and ten per week. Side effects are similar to the preceding Ergomar discussion, with nausea and nervousness being common. Because of the caffeine, anxiety or nervousness is more common with Cafergot pills than with Ergomar. The same precautions discussed above in the Ergomar section also apply to Cafergot.

**Compounded Cafergot Suppositories (only compounded available)** These are less convenient but much more effective than the pills. Cafergot suppositories contain 2 mg of ergotamine tartrate and 100 mg of caffeine. The primary side effects are nausea and anxiety. The initial dose is one third or one half of a suppository and then the dose is titrated up or down, depending on the patient's response. The dose may be repeated after 1 h, up to a maximum of two suppositories per day and five per week. Some patients find that as little as one fifth of a suppository is all that they require. Side effects of Cafergot suppositories are the same as those of Cafergot pills. Nausea and anxiety always are limiting factors in the use of ergots.

**Compounded Cafergot PB Suppositories (only compounded available)** These are similar but more effective than plain Cafergot suppositories. Cafergot PB contains 2 mg of ergotamine tartrate, 100 mg of caffeine, 60 mg of sodium pentobarbital, and 0.25 mg of 1-alkaloids of belladonna. Dosage is the same as for the plain Cafergot suppositories. Side effects are decreased, with less nausea and nervousness. Sedation may be a problem, however.

**Dihydroergotamine** This is different from the other ergots in that it is primarily a venoconstrictor rather than an arterial constrictor. Since 1945, there have been relatively few serious side effects reported. DHE is available as an intramuscular (IM) or subcutaneous (SQ) injection or as a nasal spray (Migranal®). The usual dose is 1 mg IM or SQ, or one spray in each nostril to be followed in 10–20 min by one further spray of Migranal in each nostril. Side effects tend to be minimal with DHE, but nausea, a heat or flushed sensation, nasal stuffiness from the spray, or leg cramps may occur. Occasionally, chest heaviness is also seen. While DHE is not as effective as sumatriptan for cluster headache, DHE at times is the best alternative in patients who may be at some risk for cardiac disease. However, if patients have major risk factors such as uncontrolled HTN or have known atherosclerotic heart disease, then DHE must be avoided. The usual maximum is three injections per day or two nasal sprays in each nostril per day. A new inhaled form of DHE is expected to be approved shortly. The inhaled form will have better efficacy than the Migranal spray, but not as effective as the injections.

**Cambia** Cambia is a powdered form of diclofenac potassium, 50 mg. Cambia is *only* officially Food and Drug Administration (FDA) approved for migraine, not for cluster. The usual dose is one packet (with water, or apple juice) every 2 or 3 h as needed. Gastrointestinal (GI) side effects may limit use. Cambia may be combined with a triptan. Cambia has a quicker onset of action than tablets of nonsteroidal anti-inflammatory drugs (NSAIDs).

**Ketorolac Nasal Spray (Sprix) or Ketorolac Injections** Sprix is a nasal spray of ketorolac, faster acting than tablets but not as powerful as the injections. Sprix is relatively well tolerated; the usual side effects include a feeling of burning in the throat, and GI side effects. The ketorolac injections, 30 or 60 mg, are effective for many migraine and cluster sufferers. GI and renal concerns limit use with ketorolac. Ketorolac should be limited to six doses per week.

The abortive analgesic medications include, among others, the following:

- Extra Strength Excedrin®
- Butalbital compounds (Fiorinal®, Fioricet, Esgic®, Phrenilin: all are available as generic)
- Opioids

In general, we do not want to have cluster patients rely on butalbital or opioids. However, in some refractory patients the pain is so severe and the other therapies are ineffective, justifying the use of butalbital or opioids. The milder approaches, such as Excedrin, should be utilized first, then the butalbital compounds or opioids. While rebound or withdrawal headache is less of a concern with cluster than migraine, we still must try and limit the abortives. At times, this is not an easy task.

**Lidocaine Spray** Used as a 4 % lidocaine solution, the spray has been used since the mid-1980s for cluster headache. I have found it only mildly effective for most patients and almost never adequate by itself. However, intranasal lidocaine does provide sufficient relief to warrant its use. Lidocaine is very safe, with minimal side effects. When used in conjunction with ice and one of the first-line abortives, the lidocaine spray may add 10–30 % relief.

I put 4 % topical lidocaine in a plastic nasal spray bottle. The patient is then instructed to lie in the supine position, extend their head back 30–45°, turn the head toward the side of the pain, and spray two or three sprays of the lidocaine intranasally. This may be repeated, but I usually limit the lidocaine sprays to six or eight in a 24-h period. If the nasal passage is blocked, several drops of 0.5 % phenylephrine may be used prior to the lidocaine.

Alternatively to the spray bottle, 1 ml of 4 % topical lidocaine may be slowly dropped, via a dropper, into the nostril on the side of the pain. Side effects are minimal and may include numbness in the throat or, rarely, nervousness or tachycardia. Note this is an update of article originally published in *Practical Pain Management*, Vol. 10, July 2010, and Vol. 11, March 2011.

## Preventive Therapy for Cluster Headaches

### *Preventive Medications (See Table 4.2)*

Each cluster patient is unique, with a number of variables determining where we go with medications If a patient has a short episodic cycle, we may just use abortives, or cortisone plus abortives. For longer cycles, we want to initiate one of the usual preventives, such as verapamil. Chronic cluster patients usually require daily medication for most of the year. Most often, we use cortisone (usually prednisone) for a short period of time, while initiating another preventive, such as verapamil. Prednisone, while usually very effective, should be limited; we want to minimize cortisone side effects. There is some evidence that cluster sufferers may be slightly more prone than others to femoral head necrosis from cortisone.

Comorbidities often determine where we go with medications. If a cluster sufferer is older, smokes, has HTN, and reflux, we will be limited as to our medications. Age, GI problems, psychiatric conditions, and previous reactions to medications all contribute to our medication decisions. For those with chronic clusters, we want to utilize medications that have minimal long-term side effects. Table 4.2 summarizes the usual preventive approaches to preventing cluster headaches. For quick relief, occipital injections with bupivacaine and/or cortisone may be effective. Frontally, the SPG blocks, with bupivacaine, often are helpful for frontal chronic migraine, and cluster headache. They are done via the newer Tx360 device, or the SphenoCath device. SPG blocks, with one of these devices, are very safe, and only take minutes to administer.

**Table 4.2** Common preventive medications for cluster headaches

| Class/agent | Dosage | Side effects | Comments |
|---|---|---|---|
| Corticosteroid: Prednisone | 20–40 mg/day for 3–6 days, then taper off over 4–8 days | Corticosteroids have many adverse effects. When used for short periods of time, the most common side effects are insomnia, gastrointestinal (GI) upset, and anxiety. Serious adverse events have occurred with even short courses of corticosteroids | Very effective for cluster headache, cortisone is used primarily for episodic cluster headaches. It is given for 1–2 week duration during the peak of the cluster series. Additional cortisone may be given later in the cycle, when the cluster headaches increase. Higher doses may be needed when the cluster cycle is peaking in intensity. Due to adverse side effects, it is very important to minimize the use of cortisone |
| Calcium channel blockers: Verapamil ER | At onset of headache, 240 mg/day or bid—maximum dose 480 mg/day | Constipation. Electrocardiogram (ECG) should be performed because of possible cardiac abnormalities when higher doses are used | Very effective in episodic and chronic cluster headaches. Often initiated at the onset of the headache, in conjunction with cortisone. Verapamil is then continued while the cortisone is tapered and then stopped. Because of its efficacy and minimal side effects, verapamil is a mainstay of cluster headache prevention |
| Lithium | 300–900 mg/day | Well tolerated at low doses; drowsiness, mood swings, nausea, tremor and diarrhea may occur | Helpful for chronic cluster, and to a lesser degree, episodic cluster headaches. It may be combined with verapamil and/or cortisone. Blood tests need to be performed to assess kidney and thyroid function |
| Nonsteroidal anti-inflammatory agents (NSAIDS): indomethacin | Indomethacin: 25 mg once or bid; up to 75 mg bid or tid | GI side effects may limit use | Powerful NSAID, indomethacin can be helpful for some cluster headache patients |
| Antiepileptic agents: Sodium valproate | 500–1500 mg/day | May cause weight gain, fatigue, and GI upset, among other side effects | Valproate and topiramate are occasionally effective against cluster headaches. They are the mainstay of treatment against migraines, but less effective against cluster headaches |

**Table 4.2** (continued)

| Class/agent | Dosage | Side effects | Comments |
|---|---|---|---|
| Topiramate | 50–200 mg/day | Does not cause weight gain, but cognitive side effects may limit use | – |
| Botulinum toxin A injection (only occasionally used; off label for cluster headache; not as effective as for chronic migraine) | 50–200 units | Safe, usually no adverse effects; may cause eye droop, or (rarely) generalized weakness | Botulinum toxin type A FDA-approved for chronic migraine. While the injections are not as effective for cluster headaches, they do help in some patients |
| Occipital injection: Corticosteroid and/or bupivacaine | Triamcinolone: 20–40 mg Other forms of injectable steroid have also been utilized. Bupivacaine, 2–5 ml (usually 0.5 %) | Steroid injection: local site reaction, or systemic corticosteroid effects (see above) | May decrease cluster headache occurrence for up to 4 weeks |
| Sphenopalatine ganglion nerve blocks (Allevio or Tianx360 or SphenoCath devices) | Bupivacaine (or lidocaine) | Bupivacaine: allergic reactions may occur (rare) | May decrease cluster headache occurrence for up to 2 weeks |

**Refractory Clusters:** For those cluster sufferers who have not found relief with the usual ministrations, a number of approaches have been utilized. Unfortunately, because of the small numbers in limited studies, evidence is lacking for many refractory approaches. These approaches include: stimulants (methylphenidate, mixed amphetamine salts), melatonin, testosterone, SPG blocks, daily opioids, daily triptans (used as a preventive), daily ergots (rarely used), botulinum toxin, and psilocybin, among others. There are several cluster headache support groups, such as Clusterbusters. Clusterbusters runs an excellent annual meeting of cluster headache sufferers.

I have found daily triptans (usually one at night, as a preventive) to be helpful for some patients. The longer-acting triptans, frovatriptan and naratriptan, are usually used for use on a daily basis. SPG blocks are easy to administer with the newer devices (Tx360, Allevio, and SphenoCath), and used 2–4 times weekly they can be very helpful. For some refractory chronic clusters, the implantable ATI SPG stimulator may be very helpful; this is being utilized at several centers in Europe, and studies are ongoing in the USA. As a last resort, opioids may at least alleviate some of the suffering. Psilocybin (illegal in the USA; we cannot advocate its use) has had some research behind it, and has been helpful for some patients.

## *Sample Case History*

Richard is a 40-year-old man with a history of 4-week long cycles of cluster headaches, occurring once a year in the fall. The headaches began when he was 35. The cluster period begins slowly, increasing over 1 week's time and reaching a peak where Richard has two or three severe attacks per day. These occur during the night from 10 p.m. to 3 a.m. Each cluster attack lasts from 40 to 90 min, and the pain is severe. The headache is always on the right side, and is accompanied by eye tearing and nasal congestion.

## *Treatment Plan*

Richard visits our office during the first week into his 4-week headache series. The headaches are increasing in intensity and he is miserable from the pain. At this point, we want to put Richard on a prophylactic regimen, and give him an abortive to help ease the acute attack. We decide to use prednisone, one 20-mg tablet in the morning and another with dinner (40 mg/day) for 4 days. We will reduce this to 20 mg/day after the first 4 days, and then to 10 mg/day after another 6 days. We will then taper off the prednisone entirely over the next 4–6 days.

Limiting the amount of corticosteroids is important for two reasons: (1) serious side effects are decreased and (2) if necessary, we may want to utilize additional prednisone later in the cluster series. If the patient has been on a high dose of steroids for 3 weeks, we cannot use more corticosteroid. In contrast, by keeping the amount to a minimum, we are able to use steroids later in the cluster period. Cluster sufferers may be more prone to femoral head necrosis with the use of corticosteroids.

With the prednisone, we begin a slow release form of verapamil. This is started at 240 mg/day; we may eventually increase to two doses per day, which is generally the maximum (480 mg/day). As the prednisone dose is decreased, and the patient is weaned off the medication, it is hoped that the verapamil will have taken effect.

The use of oxygen as an abortive is discussed with Richard, but he prefers to wait. We give him sumatriptan tablets, 100 mg, as he is reluctant to self-inject sumatriptan. Richard is also instructed to apply ice to the areas of pain. (See Table 4.2 for list of the most common preventative agents prescribed for cluster headaches.)

## *Results*

Six days later, Richard calls the office. He has had 5 very good days, but as the prednisone is being decreased, the headaches are becoming more severe. Sumatriptan tablets do not help; last night, he had 90 min of extremely intense pain. At this point, we convince Richard to try oxygen, at 12–15 L/min, as needed, and he rents a tank. Richard also is given sumatriptan injections, 4 mg.

We continue the original plan of decreasing prednisone, and we increase the dose of verapamil to 480 mg/day. We will monitor Richard's blood pressure. He now has oxygen and sumatriptan injections available as abortive agents; adding lithium or valproate are considerations, as is indomethacin.

I see Richard 4 days later. He is now in his third week of clusters, and by his previous pattern, has 1–2 weeks left in the cycle. However, at times a cluster period may exceed the previous one in length, and extended cluster periods of up to several months do occur. Richard states that the oxygen does help his headaches.

The clusters are less severe, but still occur regularly twice at night. Sumatriptan injections stop the attacks within 10 min of administration. The verapamil may be having some effect as well. He is down to 20 mg/day of prednisone, and we decide to taper off the dose over the next 4 days. If the headaches increase dramatically, he could return to the prednisone.

Six days later, the headaches are gone, and after a week without headaches, Richard is tapered off the verapamil over the course of 6 days. If the headaches were to return during those 6 days, we would immediately increase the dose of verapamil to the maximum of 480 mg, and consider using prednisone again.

## *Discussion*

It is important to chart which medications are most effective for treating a patient's cluster headaches, so as to be ready to use them for the next cluster series. I usually write the plan for the next series in the patient's chart, and inform the patient of the plan.

In Richard's case, we would use oxygen as an abortive, with injections of sumatriptan. As a preventive, he would be given verapamil, increasing to 480 mg/day, and approximately 2 weeks of prednisone. Instead of the injections, zolmitriptan (Zomig) nasal spray would be a consideration, and occipital nerve blocks are a reasonable possibility. SPG blocks are a strong consideration. Other preventives would include lithium, indomethacin, sodium valproate, or topiramate.

Most patients with cluster headaches are prescribed both preventative and abortive therapies. Compared to migraine management, we have relatively few medications that are effective for the treatment of cluster headaches. In order to minimize the use of corticosteroids, it is important to initiate preventive medications early in the cluster cycle. For the typical episodic cluster cycle, we begin medication with the onset of the cluster, and discontinue all medication shortly after the cycle ends. There is no demonstrated utility in continuing medication after the episodic cycle ends. Note this is an updated version of articles originally appearing in *Practical Pain Management*.

**Legal Note** This discussion is not prescriptive; all medications have side effects, and should not be used without informed consent and a discussion between the patient and physician.

# Chapter 5
# Psychological Comorbidities

## Anxiety in a Headache Patient

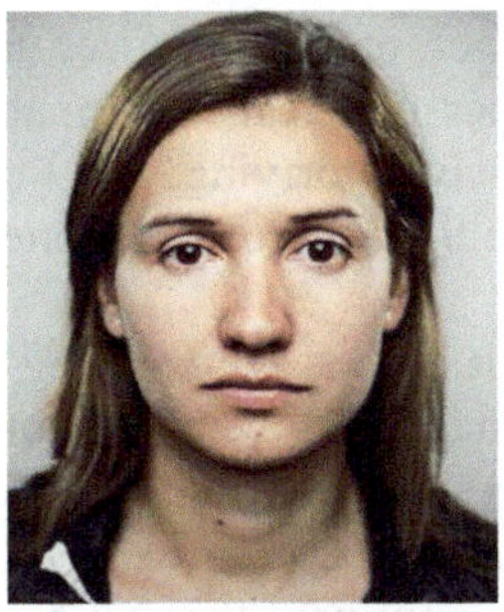

Caitlin is a 27-year-old woman with a history of migraines and anxiety. She began having separation anxiety at age 5. The patient can remember hanging onto her mother's leg "for dear life" on the first day of kindergarten. Later, at 9 years of age, symptoms of obsessive–compulsive disorder (OCD) began; these included intrusive thoughts, an aversion to germs, and the compulsion to touch everything "equally on both sides." These symptoms waxed and waned over time. By age 15, Caitlin suffered from generalized anxiety disorder (GAD), with intense worrying and feeling "keyed up." The anxiety would, at times, trigger a migraine. Additionally, when Caitlin's headaches were worse, her anxiety also increased.

Over the years, Caitlin found yoga, Pilates, and exercise to be helpful in managing her anxiety. She also noted that cognitive-behavioral psychotherapy was very useful. Biofeedback was "not for her," but she was able to use breathing techniques to calm herself down. As far as medications, she was prescribed fluoxetine (Prozac) and later switched to escitalopram (Lexapro). The selective serotonin reuptake

---

In headache patients, anxiety may increase pain while pain may fuel anxiety.Note: this is an updated version of an article that originally appeared in *Practical pain Management* in 2012.



L. Robbins, *Advanced Headache Therapy,* DOI 10.1007/978-3-319-13899-2_5

inhibitor (SSRI) helped her anxiety, but not the migraines. She did take alprazolam (Xanax) for acute, severe anxiety.

She was switched to serotonin norepinephrine reuptake inhibitors (SNRIs), starting with duloxetine (Cymbalta) and then desvenlafaxine (Pristiq). These agents helped to treat the anxiety and, to a lesser extent, the migraines. A course of gabapentin did not help the anxiety or the headaches. Caitlin feels that with therapy and medications, she remains anxious but is significantly improved.

Caitlin's history is fairly typical; anxiety may change over time, both in form and in severity. The search for effective medications may take time, as there is no accurate predictor of who will do well with what medication.

## *What Is Anxiety?*

Anxiety is a necessary and universal emotion. With anxiety that originates from a real or perceived threat of danger, one experiences an increase in heart rate, blood pressure, diaphoresis, and other physical accompaniments to anxiety. At times, anxiety comes across as excessive worrying, and this leads to avoidant behavior. Hypervigilance is an excessive focusing of one's attention on a possible danger or perceived danger.

When we think of anxiety, it is usually revolving around a problem or threat in the future. Fear, on the other hand, can be a very intense emotional reaction to a danger or threat that is in the present. We react to immediate dangers with the "fight-or-flight" response. Fear and anxiety, to some extent, are crucial for our existence. Fear allows us to escape from imminent threats; anxiety allows us to prepare for future problems. Anxiety, at least in low or moderate amounts, helps motivate many people to achieve. When someone crosses from moderate to high anxiety, it usually will interfere with the ability to perform.

The triggers for fear and anxiety may be internal or external. With internal triggers, one may have panic attacks that accelerate, feeding on themselves, in part because the associated tachycardia can convey the message that a serious physical problem is imminent. External triggers involve situations that may trigger phobias, or severe anxiety. These may include social situations, crowded or closed-in spaces, tests or other performances, etc. This leads to avoidant behavior, as anxious patients will tend to avoid those situations.

## *Types of Anxiety*

### Separation Anxiety Disorder

Patients with separation anxiety disorder have a fear of leaving a close relationship, such as the parent or home situation. Separation anxiety begins in childhood, and may or may not continue later on in life. It may manifest itself for the first time in kindergarten, with the child hanging onto the mother. Approximately, 5 % of the adult population has had the symptoms of separation anxiety. Separation anxiety may morph into a panic disorder or GAD.

### Panic Disorder

Panic attacks occur with a number of physical symptoms that may include feelings of choking, trembling, diaphoresis, racing heart, shortness of breath, chest pain, fears of losing control or dying, numbness, chills or flushing, dizziness, lightheadedness, or fainting. Panic attacks usually reach their peak quickly, and last minutes to 1 or 2 h. While they may be triggered by situations such as having to speak in public, they often occur without any obvious external trigger. Panic attacks may occur with agoraphobia, which involves a fear of situations where escape is not easy. These include public places and crowds, public transportation, highway driving, being on a bridge, or in an elevator or other enclosed space, being far from home or alone, or being stuck at a party. Agoraphobia such as this may occur without panic disorder.

### Generalized Anxiety Disorder

GAD involves excessive worrying, which may be about school, work, family, health, finances, or the outside world. With GAD, most people worry on a daily basis, not just occasionally. To diagnose GAD, the worrying must have been present for at least 6 months. People with GAD do not worry about just one facet of life, but many things. The worry becomes completely out of proportion to the significance of the problems. They also feel the physical aspects of anxiety, such as feeling "keyed up," having concentration problems, insomnia, irritability, anger, or fatigue. Approximately, 5–6% of the population suffers from GAD. It is more common in women than in men.

### Social Anxiety Disorder

Social anxiety disorder is common during adolescence, particularly with the onset of dating, parties, and other social events. It may persist into the adult years. Public speaking is difficult for those with Social anxiety disorder, and this and other triggers can lead to avoidant behavior. Approximately 12% of the population experiences Social anxiety disorder at some point.

### Obsessive–Compulsive Disorder

OCD often has an onset in early adolescence. The obsessions are intrusive, and distressing thoughts become focused on one or more concerns: germs or other contaminants, a need to have things arranged perfectly, a fear of hurting someone close, somatic (body) obsessions, hoarding, or sexual or religious obsessions. Compulsions are actions that reduce the person's anxiety somewhat, and are triggered by the obsessions. Compulsions can take the form of obsessive checking (particularly things like locks or a stove), repeated cleaning routines, repetition of words, prayers or actions, counting, or arranging objects over and over. As with most anxiety symptoms, OCD may wax and wane over time.

## *Posttraumatic Stress Disorder*

This occurs following one or repeated traumas, such as abuse of various types, a serious accident, combat, being in a fire, etc. Symptoms of posttraumatic stress disorder (PTSD) include reliving the trauma through flashbacks or nightmares, and subsequent avoidance of certain situations. PTSD may lead to feeling detached, or having amnesia for certain parts of the trauma. Hypervigilance may occur, with increased arousal and insomnia, concentration problems, anger, and a marked startle response. Approximately, 6–7 % of the population has had PTSD.

## *The Limbic System*

A propensity to anxiety is a physical, inherited illness, as is migraine. It is not psychological! By viewing certain key structures in the brain, such as the amygdala, one can almost predict who has anxiety. Even at age 5, in a child with separation anxiety, the amygdala is larger than normal and fires more often. Anxiety could almost be termed "the overactive amygdala syndrome."

The amygdala is part of the larger limbic system, which includes the thalamus, hippocampus, hypothalamus, along with the anterior cingulate gyrus and the orbitofrontal cortex. The amygdala warns of incoming dangers, after processing multiple incoming sensory inputs. Amygdala connections are vast, with direct connections to:

1. The hypothalamus, triggering fight-or-flight responses
2. The locus ceruleus (in the pons), increasing the output of norepinephrine, with a resulting rise in blood pressure, heightened response to fear, and level of alertness
3. Various other structures, such as the periaqueductal gray matter, modulating aspects of our fear response. The amygdala regulates the tone of our emotions, and is hyperreactive in anxious patients

The hypothalamus initiates our fear response; when it overreacts, the resultant anxiety is out of proportion to the actual threat. The hypothalamus may trigger an overproduction of corticotrophin release factor, adding to the anxiety response. The thalamus is our integrating relay station, with a vital direct connection to the amygdala. The thalamus controls many brain functions, and its amygdala connection initiates our stress response. The thalamus plays a vital role in regulating sleep and eating patterns, which often are disrupted in anxious patients. The hippocampus is crucial for memory, and it holds the memories that trigger the fear response. The hippocampus is important in the development of PTSD by holding onto the traumatic memories.

## *Treatments of Anxiety in Pain Patients*

### Nonpharmaceutical Approaches

Pharmacotherapy is important in treating anxiety, but it is by no means the only treatment. For those with severe pain and psychologic comorbidities, "it takes a village" to treat a patient, which may include psychotherapists, yoga or Pilates instructors, biofeedback specialists, etc.

Taking medicine alone is considered passive coping and is not sufficient for those with severe anxiety. People are best off when they exercise regularly, and learn relaxation techniques, whether they are based in yoga, Pilates, tai chi, deep breathing, biofeedback, or meditation. We need to promote this "active coping" as a vital component of treating chronic pain and anxiety. The addition of psychotherapy, primarily cognitive/behavioral, is also important. It is vital to locate an excellent therapist, and for the patient to stick with that therapist for at least 4–6 months. While short-term therapy is better than no therapy, we believe that the ideal timeframe is 1 or more years. It takes some time to integrate the ideas of therapy into our lives. Self-help books, while somewhat useful, do not replace a great therapist; neither does talking to a close friend or relative. A great therapist can be life changing.

## *Medications for Anxiety*

### Benzodiazepines

Benzodiazepines are a well-recognized treatment for anxiety, and are best used for acute anxiety, or a panic attack. Alprazolam is the most effective benzodiazepine for panic attacks, and is best used on an "as needed" basis. The lowest effective dose should be used; usual doses are 0.25–1 mg (start with ½ or 1 of the 0.25 mg tablets) as needed. Alprazolam should be limited and the patient closely monitored for overuse. Limited quantities should be prescribed.

At times, in a minority of patients, daily benzodiazepines are warranted. The usual situation is when the patient cannot tolerate nonaddicting approaches, such as the antidepressants. For insomnia, the occasional patient will only do well with a benzodiazepine, such as clonazepam (Klonopin). Diazepam (Valium) has antianxiety and muscle relaxant properties. Patients must be warned of the dangers of overuse and of combining these agents with alcohol or opioids, as well as the difficulty patients may encounter on withdrawal. For some highly anxious patients, the only medication tolerated is a benzodiazepine.

### Antidepressants: Tricyclics

The older tricyclic antidepressants (TCAs) are more useful for certain types of pain (particularly headaches) than are the SSRIs or SNRIs. We will often use a TCA in anxious pain patients in an attempt to treat both their anxiety and migraine in order to minimize medication use. The prototype tricyclic is amitriptyline (Elavil). Amitriptyline is inexpensive, and is useful for chronic daily headache, migraine, neuropathy, fibromyalgia, etc. We recommend that clinicians start with very low doses of amitriptyline, taken at night, 5 mg (½ of a 10-mg tablet), slowly increasing to 20 or 25 mg per day. Doses may be increased to 100 mg (or more), but side effects may limit its usefulness. These include sedation, dry mouth, constipation, dizziness, weight gain, and urinary retention. Other TCAs include nortriptyline, a milder form of amitriptyline; doxepin, which has fewer side effects and is helpful for insomnia; and protriptyline (Vivactil). Protriptyline is one of the few TCAs that does not cause weight gain, but anticholinergic effects limit its use.

### Antidepressants: SSRIs and SNRIs

Because of the potential for adverse events, the newer SSRIs and SNRIs are often favored over the older TCAs. The major SSRIs differ somewhat in their side effect profile. Some patients do extremely well with one SSRI, but not with another. The most common side effects include nausea, spaciness, drowsiness or fatigue, dry mouth, anxiety, insomnia, decreased libido, impotence, asthenia, sweating, constipation, tremor, diarrhea, and anorexia. In addition, weight gain may be a major problem. In fact, weight gain and sexual side effects are the most common reason to discontinue an SSRI. Any of the SSRIs can decrease motivation.

Since many of the adverse events are dose related, one key to minimizing side effects is to begin with low doses—"start low and go slow" (Table 5.1). Minimizing the dose can, for instance, decrease the sedation or sexual side effects. Compliance is enhanced when the SSRIs are slowly titrated. The initial anxiety seen with SSRIs often abates if low enough doses are used.

At times, we will use a combination of older TCAs (usually at night) and SSRIs in the morning. One of the SNRIs, duloxetine, has several pain and GAD indications, making it a useful tool for treating the comorbid migraine patient. Table 5.2 highlights the SSRIs and SNRIs. In some patients, SSRIs actually exacerbate headaches. Fluoxetine is an inhibitor of the cytochrome P450 (CYP450) 2D6 system, and to a lesser extent, CYP450 3A4.

**Table 5.1** Keys to using antidepressants in comorbid anxiety and pain patients

| |
|---|
| Start with very low doses. This minimizes sedation and anxiety and increases compliance. If the patient is bipolar, SSRIs are best avoided. |
| If patients are warned about the initial anxiety that may occur with SSRIs |
| For most headache patients, lower doses are utilized than for severe depression |
| If one SSRI does not help or causes side effects, it is often worthwhile to try another. Patients have widely differing responses to these medications |
| Slowly withdraw patients in order to avoid withdrawal syndrome |
| If the headaches are exacerbated, discontinue the SSRI |
| Paroxetine (Paxil), fluoxetine (Prozac), and duloxetine (Cymbalta) have more drug interactions than the others. These are all cytochrome P450 2D6 inhibitors |

*SSRIs* selective serotonin reuptake inhibitors

## The Major SSRIs

### These Are More Effective for Moods than for Headaches

*Fluoxetine* (Prozac, generic) is available in 10, 20, and 40 mg pulvules; 10 mg scored tablets; or liquid (20 mg/5 mL). Prozac Weekly is a once per week capsule, equal to 20 mg daily. Fluoxetine is the prototype SSRI, having been used in tens of millions of people. Fluoxetine is a long-acting SSRI with a well-established track record. Its elimination half-life is 4–6 days, but the active metabolite, norfluoxetine, has an elimination half-life of 4–16 days. The long half-life is generally an advantage in avoiding the SSRI withdrawal syndrome. It is important to start with low doses of SSRIs; 5 or 10 mg of fluoxetine is a good starting point. Many patients report initial anxiety (or even panic) from SSRIs, and if they are on a low enough dose, they are less likely to discontinue the medication. Patients can begin with ½ a tablet of 10 mg fluoxetine. Over 4–10 days, the dose may be raised to 10 or 20 mg. The effective dose for migraine or tension headache varies widely, from 5 mg per day to 60 mg (or more). Formal studies on fluoxetine for headache prevention have yielded mediocre results. Most patients are on 20 mg daily. Milder tension-type headache often responds to low doses (10 or 20 mg). As is true with TCAs, lower doses of SSRIs are used for headache doses, sertraline is a CYP450 2D6 and 3A4 inhibitor. *Sertraline* (Zoloft, generic) is available in 25, 50, and 100 mg scored tablets. Sertraline is somewhat shorter acting; elimination half-life is 26 h of the parent drug and 62–104 h of the active metabolite. Because the half-life is shorter than with fluoxetine, patients are occasionally able to stop sertraline for 1 or 2 days and alleviate the sexual side effects. However, with the shorter half-life, withdrawal syndrome is occasionally seen with sertraline. I usually start with 25 mg, or ½ of a 25-mg tablet, and slowly increase; the average antidepressant dose is 75–150 mg, but the usual headache dose is approximately 50 mg. While many patients are on 100 mg or more for headaches, most patients are maintained on lower doses. The cost of the 50 and 100 mg tablets is approximately the same.

*Paroxetine* (Paxil, generic) is available in 10, 20, 30, and 40 mg tablets. Paxil CR (controlled release) is available in 12.5 and 25 mg doses. The elimination half-life is 21 h, with no active metabolite. Paroxetine is generally very well tolerated.

**Table 5.2** Major SSRIs and SNRIs for anxiety in pain patients

| Drug name (brand) | Formulation | Usual dosage | Comments |
|---|---|---|---|
| SSRIs | | | |
| *Citalopram* (*Celexa, generic*) | Oral tablet | ½ of a 20-mg tablet/day for 4–6 days (initial dose); may go up to 40 mg/day | Effective and well-tolerated antidepressant. Mean terminal half-life is ≈35 h; has a clean drug–drug interaction profile (i.e., cytochrome P450 enzymes). Side effect profile similar to other SSRIs |
| *Escitalopram* (*Lexapro*) | Oral tablet | ½ of a 10-mg tablet/day for 4–6 days (initial dose); limit to 30 mg/day | Well tolerated with a favorable side effect profile similar to other SSRIs. Fairly clean drug–drug interaction profile |
| *Fluoxetine* (*Prozac, others*) | Oral tablet, oral Pulvule, oral liquid | 5 or 10 mg/day for 4–10 days (initial dose); limit to 80 mg/day | Well-established, long-acting SSRI; half-life is 4–6 days—an advantage in avoiding SSRI withdrawal syndrome. Important to start with low doses so patients are less likely to discontinue the medication |
| *Paroxetine (Paxil, generic)* | Oral tablet and oral CR tablet | Oral tablet: ½ of a 10-mg tablet/day (initial dose); limit to 30 mg/day Oral CR tablet: 12.5 mg tablet/day (initial dose); limit to 25 mg/day | Well tolerated with no active metabolite and a shorter half-life of 21 h. Discontinue slowly to minimize withdrawal symptoms, which can include flu-like symptoms, malaise, dizziness, and asthenia. Adding fluoxetine may help wean patient off |
| *Sertraline (Zoloft, generic)* | Oral tablet | ½ of a 25 mg tablet/day (initial dose) Average dose for antidepressant: 75–150 mg/day. Average dose for headache: 50 mg/day | Shorter half-life (26 h). Patients can usually stop sertraline for 1–2 day and alleviate sexual side effects. Due to short half-life, withdrawal syndrome is occasionally seen |
| *Vilazodone (Viibryd); Fetzima and Brintellix are also newer antidepressants* | Oral tablet | 5 or 10 mg tablet/day (initial dose); up to 40 mg/day Fetzima: 20–80 mg daily; Brintellix: 5–20 mg daily | Newer SSRI with dual mechanism of action. Is well tolerated, and may have lower incidence of weight gain and sexual side effects |

I usually begin with ½ of a 10-mg tablet and slowly increase to 10 or 20 mg; many patients need 30–60 mg for depression. Another option is starting with 12.5 mg CR and titrate as needed to 25 mg CR. It is important to stop paroxetine slowly in order to minimize withdrawal. Paroxetine (SSRI) withdrawal consists of one to several days (and occasionally longer) of flu-like symptoms, malaise, dizziness, and asthenia. This often goes unreported to the physician. Managing the withdrawal

**Table 5.2** (continued)

| Drug name (brand) | Formulation | Usual dosage | Comments |
|---|---|---|---|
| SNRIs | | | |
| *Desvenlafaxine* (*Pristiq*) | Oral capsule | 50 mg capsule/day (initial dose); up to 100 mg/day | Highly effective and tolerable antidepressant. Useful in headache patients who have concurrent anxiety/depression. Side effects include nausea, constipation, somnolence, dry mouth, dizziness, insomnia, and agitation. At lower doses, is classified as an SSRI |
| *Duloxetine* (*Cymbalta*) | Oral capsule | 20 or 30 mg capsule/day (initial dose); 60 mg/day is usual dose for depression | Very effective antidepressant and has three FDA pain indications. May benefit both headache and anxiety/depression. Side effects include nausea, dry mouth, anxiety, fatigue, lethargy, sexual effects, and weight gain. Use with caution in patients with glaucoma |
| *Venlafaxine* (*Effexor XR, generic*) | Oral capsule | 37.5 mg capsule/day (initial dose); 75 or 150 mg/day is usual dose for depression | Highly effective and tolerable antidepressant. Useful in headache patients who have concurrent anxiety/depression. Side effects include nausea, constipation, somnolence, dry mouth, dizziness, insomnia, and agitation. At lower doses, is classified as an SSRI |

*CR* controlled release, *SNRIs* serotonin norepinephrine reuptake inhibitors, *SSRIs* selective serotonin reuptake inhibitors

can be difficult; at times, the addition of fluoxetine may help in weaning off of the short-acting SSRI. Paroxetine is a potent inhibitor of the CYP450 2D6 system and, to a lesser extent, 3A4.

*Citalopram* (Celexa, generic) is available in 20 and 40 mg tablets, which are scored. The mean terminal half-life is about 35 h. Citalopram has a clean profile with regard to CYP450 enzymes. It has been an outstanding antidepressant with a very good track record, and is well tolerated. Side effects are similar to the other SSRIs. As always, we start with low doses, half of a 20-mg tablet for 4–6 days, then progress to 20 mg per day. Withdrawal symptoms have been unusual with citalopram. Its use has mostly given way to escitalopram, but, due to its lower cost, citalopram is useful.

*Vilazodone* (Viibryd) is a newer SSRI with a dual mechanism of action. Vilazodone is well tolerated, and patients may have fewer problems with weight gain and sexual side effects. It is available in 10, 20, and 40 mg tablets. We start with ½ or one of a 10-mg tablet, and slowly increase to 20 or 40 mg.

*Escitalopram* (Lexapro) is a newer, more selective version of citalopram and has been fairly well tolerated. It is metabolized primarily by the liver. Escitalopram has a favorable side effect profile, but side effects are similar to the other SSRIs. Escitalopram is available in 10 and 20 mg tablets. We start with ½ of the 10-mg tablet for 4–6 days, and then increase to 10 mg daily. Withdrawal symptoms are relatively unusual with escitalopram; it is fairly clean as far as drug interactions. Escitalopram has risen to be one of the most prescribed antidepressants in the USA.

## *The Major SNRIs*

*Venlafaxine* (Effexor XR) and *Desvenlafaxine* (Pristiq) are major SNRIs. The long-acting venlafaxine is available in 37.5, 75, and 150 mg doses. Venlafaxine has been an outstanding antidepressant because of efficacy and tolerability. A generic is available, but does not consistently work as well. Desvenlafaxine is a newer form of venlafaxine, which is very well tolerated. It is available in 50 and 100 mg doses, and is usually started at 50 mg; the final dose ranges from 50 to 100 mg per day.

Basically, venlafaxine and desvenlafaxine are SSRIs at low doses; at higher doses, levels of norepinephrine, rather than dopamine, are affected. They are very well tolerated, with less weight gain and sexual side effects than some of the other antidepressants. Venlafaxine has few interactions with CYP450 enzymes, rendering it a fairly clean medication. We usually begin with 37.5 mg and progress to 75 mg, with a typical dose in headache patients being 75 or 150 mg. Effexor XR is particularly well tolerated. It is very useful in headache patients who have concurrent anxiety and depression. Sustained elevation in blood pressure may occur at higher doses, particularly 250 mg or more per day. The lower doses have not increased blood pressure. While headache is a potential side effect of venlafaxine and desvenlafaxine, it has been no more so than the rate of placebo in studies. Nausea, constipation, somnolence, dry mouth, dizziness, insomnia, and agitation are seen more than in placebo. However, if doses remain low, venlafaxine and desvenlafaxine are well tolerated. While venlafaxine and desvenlafaxine are less effective than TCAs for pain or headache, their efficacy in anxiety and depression, and their tolerability, render them extremely useful medications.

*Duloxetine* (Cymbalta) has three Food and Drug Administration (FDA) pain indications, and is a very effective antidepressant. Duloxetine increases both serotonin and norepinephrine. It is available in 20, 30, and 60 mg capsules. Duloxetine may be helpful for headache, as well as for anxiety/depression. The usual dose is 60 mg daily for depression; starting dose is 20 or 30 mg, increasing over several days to weeks. Side effects include, among others, nausea, dry mouth, anxiety, fatigue, lethargy, sexual effects, and weight gain. Use with caution in patients with glaucoma. Duloxetine is a moderate CYP450 2D6 inhibitor. It has been much more effective for moods (including anxiety and depression) than for pain.

### Newer Antidepressants

Fetzima and Brintellix are relatively new; Fetzima is unusual in that it has more norepinephrine activity than the typical SNRI (more norepi than serotonin); this may be useful for avoiding fatigue and weight gain, but it may be more activating (norepi is activating, serotonin more calming). Brintellix has unusual 5HT-7 properties; the jury is out as to the place both of these newer medications will have in treating anxiety.

### Miscellaneous Medications

In addition to antidepressants and benzodiazepines, various other medications are useful on occasion. For those migraine patients on the bipolar spectrum, antipsychotic medications, such as quetiapine (Seroquel) and aripiprazole (Abilify), are often used. These two medications can be particularly helpful for the management of anxiety and depression. Certain anticonvulsant agents may be of benefit. Gabapentin increases the neurotransmitter γ-aminobutyric acid (GABA), which calms the brain. Gabapentin may decrease certain types of pain, and some patients find it helpful for anxiety or insomnia. Pregabalin (Lyrica) is a newer form of gabapentin, and may be beneficial. Muscle relaxants are useful in some anxious patients. Preference is given to the nonaddicting muscle relaxants, such as cyclobenzaprine. These may be helpful for associated insomnia.

## *Conclusion*

Anxiety is commonly encountered in pain and headache patients. Like migraine, anxiety is an inherited physical condition. In headache patients, pain may fuel anxiety, and anxiety may increase the pain. With medications, the antidepressants remain the mainstay of preventive treatment; the benzodiazepines are used sparingly. A variety of nonmedicine approaches should also be used in treatment, such as psychotherapy, yoga, exercise, etc. For quality of life, it is crucial to treat anxiety and other psychiatric comorbidities in addition to treating the pain. Note this is an update of an article originally published in *PPM*, Vol. 12, May, 2012.

## Attention-Deficit Hyperactivity Disorder and Patients with Pain

A growing number of patients with chronic pain are presenting with attention-deficit hyperactivity disorder (ADHD). Clinicians need to understand how the disorder is diagnosed in adults, as well as how to balance various medications required to treat both ADHD and pain.

Along with anxiety and depression, ADHD is a common comorbidity among patients with chronic pain. Although most commonly diagnosed in childhood, ADHD is seen in approximately 4.7 % of adults [7].

ADHD has become a well-recognized and validated syndrome, known for the havoc it can create in patients' lives. The public is increasingly aware of ADHD, and more of our patients arrive at the clinic with that diagnosis. The current criteria relate primarily to children and adolescents and are not entirely applicable to an adult population. Because more patients carry the diagnosis and are on ADHD medications (primarily stimulants), it is important for pain physicians to be aware of the consequences of the disorder. In addition, it is helpful to be aware of interactions between ADHD and pain medications.

### *Diagnosis of ADHD in Adults*

The diagnosis of ADHD includes the patient's history along with corroborating evidence: educational records and history, family or significant other's input, and so forth. In my experience, most patients who carry the diagnosis of ADHD from childhood have been correctly diagnosed; although there is occasional overdiagnosis of ADHD, underdiagnosis remains more prevalent.

The standard criteria for the diagnosis of ADHD require that the symptoms have lasted for at least 6 months [4]. One objective test that we have found useful is the Adult Self-Report Scale (ASRS) [14], which is an 18-item questionnaire. The first nine questions relate to attention, the remaining nine to hyperactivity. Using the first nine questions gives the clinician an easy screen for ADHD and requires only minutes to administer. The attention portion of the ASRS gives a score of 0–36, with 36 being the most severe. This scale or similar ones, along with the clinical and educational histories, helps to determine the diagnosis.

An important question to ask the patient is, "How difficult is it for you to do boring tasks?" People with ADHD have great difficulty with boring material. To aid the diagnosis, I often have the patient read books or other materials on adult ADHD so that they can provide better-informed input into the diagnosis.

The three primary features of ADHD (attention, hyperactivity, and impulsivity) do change over time. As patients approach adulthood, hyperactivity often decreases, whereas impulsivity may cause more problems for adults than for children. Therefore, using hyperactivity as a measure of ADHD may not be valid in adulthood; many children and adolescents "lose" the "H" (hyperactive) portion of ADHD and present as the inattentive type.

ADHD adversely affects adults in their family and work life; these are not addressed by the current criteria. The age of onset is usually by age 7 but not always. Some patients have a somewhat older age of onset for ADHD symptoms.

In children, parents' and teachers' input is crucial. In adults, we often utilize the patient's recall for assessment in addition to asking someone who knows the person well. There are pitfalls in assessing adults; for example, we must not compare the patient with a high-functioning, high-IQ peer group, but rather with normal or average people. In addition, particularly in college students, the desire to excel on examinations or improve scores does not qualify them to be diagnosed as having ADHD.

Mood disorders may cause an attention/concentration problem in adults, leading to an inappropriate diagnosis of ADHD. However, most patients with ADHD do have associated psychiatric comorbidities, such as anxiety or depression. Many who fit on the bipolar spectrum can have concurrent ADHD. It is important to assess for all of these conditions.

## *ADHD and Impairment*

Adult patients with ADHD are often impaired in several categories. They may have done poorly in school, leading to problems with their work and career. Home life is adversely affected, with problems accomplishing daily responsibilities. Relationships are negatively affected by ADHD, and family life often falls apart as a result. The severity of childhood/teen ADHD is an accurate predictor of impairment as an adult. Young children who are constantly restless and cannot wait their turn in line, for example, often show more impairment as young adults. ADHD increases the likelihood of driving accidents and also of drug or alcohol abuse. It is probably not true that ADHD allows one to excel in certain areas; the evidence speaks more for impairment than for any positive outcome for those with ADHD, particularly if it is not treated.

The associated psychiatric comorbidities add to impairment, particularly if they are not treated. These include anxiety, depression, bipolar depression, and substance abuse.

The evidence is strong for treating ADHD. Compared with treated patients, untreated ADHD greatly increases the risk, at age 20–25, for drug abuse, accidents, joblessness, and jail. The clinical stakes for under-recognizing and undertreating ADHD are enormous. If impulsivity does not improve by the early 20s, it is a poor prognostic indicator for how the patient will do over time.

## ADHD and the Patient With Pain

ADHD complicates the lives of patients with pain. The patient struggles with functional impairment due to pain, and ADHD adds to this dysfunction. Education often suffers because of pain; students take longer to complete their degree, and the addition of the negative impact of ADHD can make completion impossible. Family life is adversely affected, as spouses may tire of the burden of pain complaints, along with the various ADHD symptoms. Chronic pain often leads to joblessness or underperforming at work; ADHD only accentuates this problem. In a patient with chronic pain and ADHD and, for instance, anxiety and depression, we commonly encounter a person who is underfunctioning in a number of areas.

## ADHD Medications

The "first-line" medications for ADHD are stimulants [13,24, 25]. The most commonly used stimulants include methylphenidate (Concerta, Ritalin, Ritalin LA, Focalin, and others: generics available), dextroamphetamine (Dexedrine, others: generics available), amphetamine and dextroamphetamine (Adderall, Adderall XR: generic available for these), and lisdexamfetamine (Vyvanse). The longer-acting forms are Adderall XR, Vyvanse, Ritalin LA, Focalin XR, Daytrana, and Concerta. Side effects of these agents include, among others, anxiety, insomnia, tachycardia, and, occasionally, increased headache. The stimulants have mild analgesic effects and in some may be an adjunct for the pain. In addition, some patients with depression find that the stimulants act as an adjunct for the depression, whereas in others they may actually exacerbate depression. Fatigue is a common comorbidity encountered in patients with pain, and stimulants may help patients' energy level during the day. In addition, the anorexiant effects are beneficial for some patients with pain, as obesity and weight gain are commonly encountered among these patients.

The stimulants may improve attention, energy level, pain, and depression as well as decrease appetite. However, many patients cannot tolerate them because of adverse effects. In addition, patients with pain are usually on various medications, with possible interactions. For instance, patients with pain often are taking antidepressants, with resulting tachycardia when combined with stimulants. When patients with pain are utilizing daily opioids, adding a stimulant contributes another potentially addicting medication. Fortunately, addiction to stimulants among adults with ADHD is uncommon.

When stimulants are not appropriate or not tolerated, there are various "second-line" medications for ADHD. The $\alpha_2$-adrenergic agonists (guanfacine ER [Intuniv], clonidine [Kapvay]) are primarily utilized in children and adolescents. Various antidepressants have been successfully used for ADHD. These include the older tricyclics (desipramine, nortriptyline) as well as bupropion. These may be appropriate with concurrent anxiety or depression. Atomoxetine (Strattera), an

SNRI, is used as a second-line medication for ADHD and is very similar to the tricyclic desipramine, which also increases norepinephrine. Although these medications are not as effective as the stimulants, they offer several benefits. These include the advantage of not being addictive, and, when used as once-daily medications, they are longer acting.

### *Nonmedication Treatments*

In addition to medications, we often refer patients to psychotherapy. Although therapy does not improve attention itself, the patient benefits in a number of ways. These include help with associated anxiety/depression, family life, relationships, organization, and work life. A good therapist who is acquainted with pain and ADHD can play a crucial role in improving functioning and quality of life.

It is important to work on sleep issues and diet. In addition, as with almost all patients, we supplement with at least 2000 units of vitamin $D_3$. We stress the role of exercise, advising patients to try to build up to 20–30 min daily on average.

### *Conclusion*

ADHD is commonly encountered, seen in 4.7 % of adults. The various symptoms complicate the lives of patients with pain. The clinical stakes for not recognizing ADHD are enormous; patients often underperform at work, have poor family relationships, and are at increased risk for substance abuse. Treatment with medications, primarily stimulants, improves quality of life and functioning. In addition, psychotherapy plays a role, as does stressing the role of sleep, nutrition, and exercise. Note this is an update of an article originally published in *Practical Pain Management*, Vol. 11, November 2011.

## Personality Disorders and the Bipolar Spectrum: Recognition and Management in a Pain Clinic Setting

### *Introduction*

Patients with moderate-to-severe personality disorders (PD) may wreak havoc on an unsuspecting medical office. It is increasingly important to recognize, limit and manage those with aggressive types of PD. Likewise, it is crucial to recognize those who fit the bipolar spectrum. In particular, the mild end of the spectrum is often missed. The clinical stakes for missing bipolar are enormous, as these patients tend to bounce from antidepressant to antidepressant, with predictably poor results. This chapter delves into recognition and management of patients whose pain treatment is complicated by psychological concerns.

## *Personality Disorders at a Clinic*

Consider the following scenario: a 28-year-old man, "Bill" presents to the pain clinic with severe low back pain. He seems angry on the first visit, and is very demanding with the front office staff. Bill is mistrustful of physicians, and openly states to the doctor, "I will go back to work when you give the right amount of drugs that help." Bill is upset with his last two health providers.

Over the next few months, the clinic bends over backwards for Bill, even though he can be abusive to the staff. Bill overuses opioids, and is manipulative. He always has a sense of entitlement. When he calls, stating, "I want to talk to Dr. Smith NOW, put me through!" the staff, out of fear, jumps, and does as he asks. The physician finds himself in a subservient position, trying to appease the patient and end the confrontations.

Bill laughs at the idea of seeing a psychotherapist, but after 9 months of treatment, Bill is suddenly blaming everything on the physician and clinic: his pain, his obesity, his sexual dysfunction. Bill threatens to sue, and reports the doctor to the state regulatory office. What happened here?

Bill will be later diagnosed as a paranoid PD. The clinic did not recognize him as such, and failed to set limits on Bill's behavior. The disruptions in the business of the clinic, the increased stress on the staff, and the monopolization of the doctor's time cannot be recovered. In the following, we discuss the features of PDs that should help with identification. Better management of the problem starts with recognition.

Approximately, 10–12 % of people have features of a PD [15]. There are a number of PDs, and some are more dangerous and difficult than others. In general, characteristics of PDs include lack of insight, poor response to psychotherapy or other therapeutic interventions, difficulty with attachments and trust, a sense of entitlement, and the creation of chaos and distress in family, friends, and coworkers. Comorbid substance abuse is common.

PDs range from mild to very severe. Patients with PDs may take on different roles: victim, rescuer, or persecutor. When they turn persecutor, they can be dangerous to the person they have set their sights on. Seeing a therapist for a long period of time, perhaps 5–7 years, helps to some degree. However, goals and expectations must be limited. The plasticity of the brain is important, as some people can improve naturally over time. The following section describes some of the more severe PD types. However, many people do not fit neatly into any of these categories, but have features of two or three PDs.

**Paranoid Personality Disorder** This type tends to be nontrusting, suspicious, and sees the world as dangerous. They may seem secretive and reluctant to confide in others. In relationships, they view themselves as being constantly mistreated. They doubt the loyalty of everybody around them, and believe they are being exploited or harmed. These patients bear severe grudges against others. Often, they become angry easily and have a sense of entitlement. Paranoid personalities can become violent and dangerous, as most spree killers are paranoid personalities. Several notorious world leaders, such as Joseph Stalin and Saddam Hussein, were most likely paranoid personalities [16].

**Antisocial Personality Disorder** These people generally have no regard for the rights of others. In demeanor, they tend to be irritable and impulsive. They are exploitative, see themselves as better or superior, and can be very opportunistic in getting what they want. Antisocials are deceitful, may steal from people around them, and often have trouble with the law. They frequently engage in fraudulent activities and make very good scam artists. For example, one may take on the role of financial savior for a church, and end up stealing everything. They generally have no remorse. Conduct disorder in a child often morphs into antisocial PD. Examples include Tony Soprano on the TV show, and, in real life, the mafia's "Dapper Don," John Gotti [16].

**Borderline Personality Disorder (BPD)** This type of personality shows instability of mood, poor self-image, and pervasive abandonment fears. There is an identity disturbance and major boundary issues. Borderlines usually demonstrate impulsiveness, and very quick shifts from depression to anxiety to irritability. There are usually chronic feelings of emptiness or severe loneliness, plus anger and temper and even suicidal behavior. Under stress, they can become somewhat paranoid. Coexisting problems with drug abuse or other addictive behaviors may occur. There are often sleep disorders with severe insomnia. Severe borderlines will react with high drama and create chaos for everybody around them. They tend to have a split view, which is, they see people as wonderful or terrible, with nothing in between. Examples include Adolph Hitler, Marilyn Monroe, and Glenn Close's character Alex, in the movie, "Fatal Attraction." Borderline personality can vary from mild to severe, and become better or worse over time. Suicide becomes more likely as patients age into their upper twenties and thirties16]. Suicide is also more common within a week of discharge from a psychiatric unit.

**Narcissistic Personality Disorder** This is less common, and is typified by a personality that sees itself as above others. The personality is grandiose, has a lack of empathy, and feels and acts self-important. There is a deep sense of entitlement. They may be very vain and constantly require admiration. They are envious, arrogant, exploitative, and can be very angry. Examples might include General George Patton, Nicole Kidman's character in the movie, "To Die For," Michael Douglas' character, Gordon Gekko, in the movie, "Wall Street [16]."

There are a number of other PDs that are not as dangerous for the people around them or for health-care providers. Even though PD characteristics may seem extreme, they are often overlooked, and health-care clinics may react by treating these patients in a dysfunctional manner. The problem begins with not recognizing the PD.

## *Pain and Personality Disorders*

One previous study on BPD concluded that BPD comorbidity with migraine is associated with increased disability from the headaches [23]. In addition, among those with BPD, there was an increase in medication overuse headache, and headaches were more pervasive. There was a higher degree of depression among those with BPD, more unscheduled visits for acute headache treatment, and a lesser chance of adequate response of headache medications. Those with BPD were more severely affected by headaches, and more inclined to be refractory to treatment [23].

Another study indicated that the incidence of BPD was increased in migraineurs [12]. My recent study of 1000 migraineurs indicated that 5.5% of patients had a moderate or severe PD [21].There is ample evidence that transformed migraine is associated with more prevalent psychopathology, including PD, than is episodic migraine. BPD itself is the mental health equivalent of chronic pain. In my experience, the two most important prognostic indicators for those with PD are impulsivity and substance abuse.

Treatment for those with PD necessitates a caring, but stern, approach. Limits must be set on physician contact, including telephone calls. No abuse of staff should be tolerated. Referral to other health-care providers, particularly mental health professionals, should be suggested. Psychotherapists and psychiatrists who are experienced with this population are vital if the patient is to be adequately managed. Many of the PD patients do not do well with traditional, insight-oriented therapy treatment, but are better managed long-term with dialectical behavioral approach. For a therapy to be beneficial, it must be consistent and long term. A psychoeducational approach may also help. Unfortunately, many PD patients will not continue in therapy, even with encouragement and support. Our therapeutic goals for the PD patient are relatively modest.

It is easy to become drawn into the drama surrounding patients with PDs, particularly those with BPD. The patient with BPD may grant his doctor power, but then subvert the therapy. An example of this would be, "Doctor, you are the greatest, only you can help me. These headaches ruin my life, … and I know that nothing is going to work!" Some physicians are able to manage these patients without becoming involved in the drama and countertransference, but most do not do well with these patients. If there are signs of a dangerous PD from the first visit or phone call to the clinic, with abuse and anger showing at times, it is better to refer the patient than to become enmeshed in the relationship.

There are risks inherent in caring for those with certain PDs. As compared to the general population, those with BPD are at increased risk for suicide, particularly as they progress into middle age. Identifiable risk factors for suicide among BPD patients include repeated hospitalizations (five or more), a recent psychiatric hospitalization, and, among adolescents, birth trauma [16]. Certain types of PD (paranoid, narcissistic, antisocial, and borderline) are more likely to become angry and vengeful with their health-care providers, resorting to lawsuits or letters to the departments of regulation. Violence may also be a threat. A PD patient often enters as a victim, then rapidly flips into the role of persecutor. Their anger becomes intently focused, creating a stressful environment for health-care workers. Setting limits and keeping careful documentation are important in these situations.

It does take a village to help a patient with a PD, just as it does to adequately treat those with severe pain. It is important to recruit others, such as mental health providers, physical therapists, biofeedback therapists, etc., to aid in the treatment.

Medications, though limited, may be beneficial for the impulsivity, aggression, self-mutilation, anxiety and depression components of PD [16]. While there are no specific medications indicated for those with PD, the Axis I symptoms are more amenable to pharmacotherapy. Antidepressants, mood stabilizers, and antipsychotics may ameliorate symptoms. Some of these medications may also lessen headache pain as well. PD patients with severe, chronic pain present additional challenges for treatment. It is important to limit and closely monitor addicting medications. Particularly with BPD, opioids and benzodiazepines are best avoided. The diagnosis of a moderate or severe PD alters both our goal and approach.

## *Bipolar Disorder*

The clinical spectrum of bipolar disorder is an evolving concept. The milder end of the spectrum often is misdiagnosed as "regular" depression. For example, the important hypomanic reaction to an antidepressant has not been included in the DSM in helping to determine bipolarity [3]. Some authors feel DSM has an inherent bias toward diagnosing PDs, rather than bipolar disorders. These biases lead to bipolar disorders being missed or underdiagnosed. The name, "bipolar," is unfair and misleading; the stigma inhibits the diagnosis. We need books and materials aimed at patients with symptoms at the milder end. When we label people with the term "bipolar," (or worse, "manic-depressive") and then prescribe "antipsychotic" drugs, it is no wonder patients resist the diagnosis.

Mania is better recognized than is hypomania (with milder bipolar features.) Symptoms of mania include euphoric mood, distractibility, flight of ideas, grandiosity, thoughtlessness or risk taking, and excessive involvement in pleasurable activities (i.e., sex, spending, gambling). Also, pressured speech, an increase in activities, excited (or irritable) energetic mood, and insomnia are indicators [2]. It is the milder end of the bipolar spectrum that tends to be missed. Look for those with persistently agitated personalities, with frequent depression or excessive energy, and those with a strong bipolar or depressive family history. They may not remember a clear hypomanic or manic episode. To aid the diagnosis, it is vital to speak with a close family member; some 40 % of hypomanias are missed if one simply talks to the patient. Mild bipolar signs include: early depression (as early as the teens), severe bouts of depression, quick onset depression, bipolar reactions to certain meds (complaints of being up all night, mind racing, etc.), agitation and anger, very high anxiety, poor response to medication, and moody personality. Sleep disorders are commonly seen. Cycles of brooding, irritable pessimism may be a manifestation of hypomania. Cyclical depression, for no clear reason, is common for bipolar depression, and may be accompanied by high anxiety. Depression is the primary problem with bipolar; it is much more pervasive than are the highs of hypomania. Left untreated, patients with bipolar often self-medicate.

As an example, consider "Jane," a 44-year-old woman with a history of depression since age 16. Her mom was depressed and an alcoholic; Jane's uncle committed suicide. In addition to the depression, Jane suffers from fibromyalgia. She tends to be irritable and angry, and self-medicates with prescription opioids and alcohol. Jane saw her family physician, who prescribed fluoxetine for her symptoms. After the first dose she was, "up all night and felt crazy, like my mind was going 95 miles an hour." So, instead of fluoxetine, sertraline was prescribed, and the same response occurred. Jane also had similar hypomania from pseudoephedrine and corticosteroids. She finally was diagnosed as bipolar II, and was placed on lamotrigine, but then developed a rash. Quetiapine was tried, but Jane seemed overly sedated. Eventually, small doses of lithium improved Jane's moodiness by 50 %, without the extreme side effects.

The therapeutic implications for not recognizing bipolarity are substantial. Patients such as Jane, when undiagnosed, are often given a number of antidepressants, with predictable hypomanic results. The TCAs appear to have the highest propensity towards triggering mania, followed by the SSRIs. Any antidepressant can provoke hypomania (or full mania) in someone who is bipolar. The best results seem to come from a combination of mood stabilizers with antidepressants, although the role of antidepressants remains controversial. The diagnosis is a crucial step, but treatment for the bipolar patient is not always easy or successful. While psychotherapy usually is helpful, many patients are reluctant to go for therapy, often due to time or money constraints.

Comorbidity of migraine with anxiety and depression is well established, both in clinically based studies and in epidemiologic samples from community populations [19]. The physiologic overlap between migraine and depression is considerable. Antidepressants or mood stabilizers help both conditions. In the vast majority of migraine patients who suffer from depression, anxiety is a complicating factor. The anxiety disorder often precedes the age of onset of migraine, with depression following afterward. It is possible that poorly controlled migraines may fuel the onset of depression, or that depression may, at times, increase headache. However, it is more likely that shared environmental and genetic factors link migraine and depression.

The relationship between bipolar illness and migraine has not been as well studied as depression and migraine. However, in several studies, bipolar I and bipolar II were found to be increased in migraineurs [8]. I previously assessed 1000 consecutive migraineurs. The results were as follows: bipolar I: 2.1 %; bipolar II: 2.4 %; cyclothymic disorder: 1.3 % bipolar disorder not otherwise specified: 2.8 %; and total bipolar spectrum: 8.6 % [22].

Other recent studies have confirmed that at least 7 % of headache patients fit into the bipolar spectrum, and 30–50 % of bipolar patients have migraines [17, 18].

Once the bipolar diagnosis is established or suspected, mood stabilizers often are very helpful for both moods and headaches. Divalproex sodium is effective for mania, hypomania, depression associated with bipolar disorder, and for headache prevention. It has been extremely well studied for these conditions and has become one of the primary migraine and chronic daily headache preventives. Lithium carbonate is underutilized; it should be used more often. One or more of the newer antiepileptics may prove to be helpful for bipolar disorders and migraine. Carbamazepine has some utility as a mood stabilizer, but not for migraine prophylaxis. Oxcarbazepine is a milder form of carbamazepine, and may be useful. Oxcarbazepine is now available in a longer-acting form, Oxtellar.

Lamotrigine is becoming one of the most commonly used mood stabilizers. It is one of the few effective medications for bipolar depression [10]. Doses must be slowly titrated, due to the one out of 2000–5000 occurrences of toxic epidermal necrolysis, or Stevens Johnson Syndrome.

The atypical antipsychotics are also used for bipolar symptoms [9]. When a mood stabilizer is effective, the underlying agitation, anger, or depression improves. Quetiapine has reasonable efficacy data. As a class, the atypicals do carry the risk of metabolic syndrome. Aripiprazole has been effective for many patients, with less sedation and metabolic issues than most of the other atypicals.

Unfortunately, the medications discussed are more effective for the manic and hypomanic symptoms. The depression often goes untreated. Bipolar patients spend the majority of their time in depression, and we need better medications for their benefit. Many patients need two to four different medications; an effective combination might be lamotrigine, lithium, and an antidepressant. Rational polypharmacy is an improvement over monotherapy in treating the various bipolar symptoms. It often takes months or years to reach the "right" balance of medications for any one individual who fits the bipolar spectrum.

## *Conclusion*

For patient care, it has become increasingly important to recognize those patients whose psychiatric problems complicate their treatment in a pain clinic. Patients with a PD are more likely to abuse drugs, file lawsuits, or abuse the staff. With PD, setting limits is vital.

For those patients with bipolar symptoms, missing the diagnosis leads to poor outcomes with medication. Instead of mood stabilizers, antidepressants tend to be wrongly utilized, usually with discouraging results for the patient. Recognition that the patient fits the bipolar spectrum is the major key.

Treating patients with chronic pain is challenging enough; for those pain patients who also have psychological comorbidities, it is vital that the psychopathology be attended to, as well as the pain. Note this is an updated version of an article that originally appeared in *Practical Pain Management*, Vol. 8, April, 2008.

## Suggested Reading

1. ADHD section at www.psychcentral.com. Accessed 2013
2. Akiskal HS (2002) Classification, diagnosis and boundaries of bipolar disorders. In: Maj M, Akiskal H, Lopez-Ibor J et al. (eds) Bipolar disorder. Wiley, London, pp 1–52
3. American Psychiatric Association (1994) Diagnostic and statistical manual of mental disorders, 4th edn. American Psychiatric Association, Washington DC
4. American Psychiatric Association (2013) Diagnostic and statistical manual of mental disorders, 5th edn. Text Revision. American Psychiatric Association, Washington DC
5. Attention Deficit Disorder Association. Support & resources. http://www.add.org. Accessed 2012
6. Barkley R (2010) Taking charge of adult ADHD. The Guilford Press, New York
7. Barkley R, Murphy K, Fischer M (2008) ADHD in adults: what the science says. The Guilford Press, New York
8. Baskin SM et al. (2006) Mood and anxiety disorders in chronic headache. Headache 46(Suppl 3):S76–S87
9. Calabrese J et al. (2005) A randomized, double-blind, placebo-controlled trail of quetiapine in the treatment of bipolar I or II depression. Am J Psychiatry 162:1351–1360
10. El-Mallakh RS, et al. (2007) Antidepressants in bipolar depression. In: El-Mallakh R, Ghaem S (eds) Bipolar depression. American Psychiatric Publishing, Washington DC, pp 149–153
11. Hallowell R, Ratey J (2011) Driven to distraction: recognizing and coping with attention deficit disorder from childhood through adulthood. Anchor Books, New York
12. Hegarty AM (1993) The prevalence of migraine in borderline personality disorder. Headache 33:271
13. Janicak P, Marder S, Pavuluri M (2010) Principles and practice of psychopharmacotherapy. 5th edn. Lippincott Williams & Wilkins, Philadelphia
14. Kessler RC, Adler L, Ames M, et al (2005) The World Health Organization adult ADHD self-report scale (ASRS): a short screening scale for use in the general population. Psychol Med 35(2):245–256
15. Lester G (2002) Personality disorders in social work and health care. Cross Country University Press, Nashville, pp 28–79
16. Lester G (2005) Borderline personality disorder. Treatment and management that works. Cross Country University Press, Nashville, pp 15–19, 24–25, 88–91
17. Low NC, et al. (2003) Prevalence, clinical correlates and treatment of migraine in bipolar disorder. Headache 64:53–59.
18. McIntyre RS, et al. (2006) The prevalence and impact of migraine headache in bipolar disorder: Results from the Canadian community health survey. Headache 46:973–982
19. Merikangas KR, et al. (1997) Comorbidity of migraine and psychiatric disorders. Neurol Clin 15:115–123
20. National Resource Center on ADHD. www.help4adhd.org. Accessed 2014

21. Robbins L (2007) Bipolar spectrum in migraine, cluster and chronic tension headache. US Neurol Dis 3(2)
22. Robbins L (2007) The prevalence of personality in migraineurs. US Neurol Dis 4(1)
23. Rothrock J et al (2007) Borderline personality disorder and migraine. Headache 47:22–26
24. Shahl S (2008) Stahl's essential psychopharmacology: neuroscientific basis and practical applications. 3rd edn. Cambridge University Press, New York
25. Stahl S (2011) The prescriber's guide. 4th edn. Cambridge University Press, New York
26. Weiss L (1992) Attention deficit disorder in adults: practical help for sufferers and their spouses. Taylor Publishing Company, Dallas

# Chapter 6
# Case Studies

## An Interactive Case History of Chronic Migraine: Part 1

*A step-by-step guide through the continued diagnosis and treatment of a refractory complex headache patient.*

New patient "Heather" (not her real name) is a 24-year-old hairdresser with migraines since age 12, which have been slowly increasing. In the past 3 years, she has endured daily headaches. Her mother and sister also have migraines. Her usual daily headache is an aching, throbbing moderate headache with photophobia. About six times per month, Heather has a moderate to severe migraine with nausea and lasting one day. She has been diagnosed with chronic migraine (CM). Triggers for her more severe migraines include weather changes, stress, and menstruation (1 day prior to her menses).

Heather has also struggled with irritable bowel syndrome (IBS) for much of her life; she has occasional constipation, but diarrhea and cramps are her usual symptoms. She has not been treated for this. She is 5'5" feet, weighs 128 lbs, and has, at times, struggled with weight gain. She does not smoke cigarettes.

Besides the daily headache, Heather has associated neck pain, with tenderness in her neck and shoulder muscles. She clenches and grinds her teeth, particularly at night while sleeping. She was prescribed diazepam, but says, "I became wired and had a bad reaction on it…"

Heather has not been on daily preventives. She consumes four Extra Strength Excedrin daily and, for her migraine, uses hydrocodone. This dampens the pain but does not help any more than 30 %.

### *Psychological Aspects*

Heather also has been diagnosed with generalized anxiety disorder and depression. She first became depressed at age 14, and has had mild to moderate chronic depression since age 18. There is a strong family history of anxiety and depression. Her grandmother was hospitalized for possible depression, and an uncle committed



L. Robbins, *Advanced Headache Therapy*, DOI 10.1007/978-3-319-13899-2_6

suicide. Heather's mom suffers from lifelong depression and has struggled with alcoholism.

Heather is chronically irritable and somewhat angry; she is prone to bouts of road rage. She has several spells a year which she describes as, "too much energy, where I don't sleep much." In certain seasons, she seems to cycle into worsening depression.

Heather was placed on fluoxetine, and she "was up all night, my mind was going too fast." She was then prescribed duloxetine (Cymbalta), and the same thing happened. Heather also becomes "wired" from certain meds, such as pseudephedrine.

In summary, Heather has moderate daily headache, with migraines six times a month, plus anxiety and depression, IBS, and neck pain.

**Outside of medication, what would you suggest for Heather?**

We need to teach Heather about regular sleep habits, not missing meals, avoiding too much caffeine, identifying stresses that may contribute to her headaches, engaging in exercise, and improving posture, etc.

In addition, a referral to a good psychotherapist would be beneficial, as would biofeedback by a skilled therapist. Psychiatric referral would be a reasonable choice as well.

For the neck pain, physical therapy may be helpful, at least as far as teaching about exercise and posture. Heather's profession as a hairdresser often will exacerbate neck pain and her headaches due to the constant arm movements. A dentist who is adept at evaluating temporomandibular disorders (TMD) may be beneficial for Heather as well.

We do not expect Heather to rush off to the psychologist, psychiatrist, physical therapist, and dentist all at once. Because of money and time, most patients carefully select which healthcare professionals they visit. However, it "takes a village" to treat a complicated pain patient and I try to refer the patient to appropriate specialists.

**What type of depression does Heather suffer from?**

We need to think about the mild end of the bipolar spectrum. According to one study, some 8.6 % of migraineurs fit into the bipolar spectrum. Heather has a number of features of bipolar disorder, including early depression (age 14), and a family history of depression, suicide, and substance abuse. Other indicators are her irritable/angry personality, cyclical depression, spells of too much energy, and poor (bipolar) reaction to certain meds (antidepressants, pseudoephedrine, diazepam). The clinical stakes for missing bipolar are enormous. Patients such as Heather tend to bounce from antidepressant to antidepressant, with predictably poor results.

**Question: What are the initial choices of preventive medication for Heather?**

Comorbidities, along with the headache characteristics, guide where we go with the headache meds. Along with the chronic daily headaches and migraines, Heather fits the mild end of the bipolar spectrum, has IBS (primarily diarrhea), neck pain, and has struggled with weight gain. All of these characteristics figure into our medication choices.

As a headache preventive, topiramate may be a good choice. It will not cause weight gain and may decrease appetite for some period of time. It may act as a mild mood stabilizer, although studies have reported both positive and negative results on topiramate as a bipolar medication. Topiramate may almost certainly exacerbate depression. We would begin with a low dose because headache patients tend to be somatic and will not tolerate large initial doses—often leading to them quit the medicine prematurely. My recommendation would be: topiramate, 25 mg, one at night for the first 6 nights, then, if tolerated, increasing to 50 mg at night. Utilizing the topiramate at night may minimize cognitive side effects and fatigue. Some patients cannot tolerate more than 25 mg of topiramate. The usual dose is 50–100 mg, although some patients do well on 25 mg, while others require 300 or 400 mg per day. The cognitive side effects of spacey feelings and memory problems often limit topiramate's use, as does the tingling sensation in fingers and toes. Primarily due to carbonic anhydrase activity, the tingling is sometimes offset via the use of potassium—either natural or in tablets/powder. There is now a longer-acting form, generic topiramate ER.

**Which abortive meds would you consider?**

Most daily headache patients have two or three abortives. They may have something for milder daily headaches, a migraine medication, and an "escape" analgesic for the severe migraine. With Heather, we do not want to go down the road of overused daily analgesics, but most patients want and need something for the daily headaches as well as for the migraine. In Heather's case, we need to emphasize that we do not want to constantly chase the headache all day, but rather use the preventive meds and nonmedication techniques to decrease the severity.

For Heather's migraines, my recommendation would be sumatriptan, 100 mg tabs. If patients have never used a triptan before, I start with a low dose the first time—such as half of a tablet. Many patients are frightened by the muscle pressure, tingling, and other side effects of the triptans, and we need to test them on a low initial dose. This will improve compliance. With the triptans and other antimigraine abortives, early intervention is crucial. There is an enormous difference between using the triptan in the first half hour and waiting an hour or more.

For Heather's nausea, we prescribe 8 mg ondansentron as this is the only antiemetic that is nonsedating. We stop the hydrocodone, except as an "escape" medication to be used on a very limited basis.

For Heather's daily headaches, we discontinue the Excedrin and instead have her use naproxen along with limited amounts of caffeine. I try and limit caffeine intake to 150 mg or, at most, 200 mg a day. She was taking 250 mg just in her daily dose of four Excedrin, with more in coffee, tea, and colas. The idea with daily abortives is to limit caffeine, use the longer-acting nonsteroidal anti-inflammatory drugs (NSAIDs) such as naproxen, and avoid addicting meds.

## *Initial Prescription*

Heather has started on topiramate as a preventive and sumatriptan as the primary abortive, with naproxen, ondansentron, and limited hydrocodone.

**What other preventive medicines are possibilities?**

When we initially see a complicated headache patient, our list of possible meds takes into account a number of factors, including all of the comorbidities: psychiatric, medical, and gastrointestinal (GI). It is helpful to note these other medicine possibilities in the chart since headache patients call often, as the meds may be ineffective or have side effects. We need to be able to easily switch meds. If you work with other physicians, they should be able to scan the chart and select another appropriate med.

With Heather, other preventive possibilities would be noted in her chart, as follows:

1. Petadolex, an excellent evidence-based natural preventive (probably the most effective "natural" preventive; we do cycle off Petadolex periodically, due to carcinogenic concerns in animals).
2. Lamotrigine, which may be helpful for her mild bipolar depression, although there is less evidence for helping the headaches.
3. Verapamil, which may help the headache, and also the diarrhea with IBS.
4. Gabapentin, which is safe, inexpensive, and easy to use; available as a longer-acting form, Gralise.
5. Sodium valproate could help her bipolar depression, but weight gain is a drawback, and we would need to warn her about risks of pregnancy; because of the major concerns with the fetus, valproate is not usually used in young women.
6. Oxcarbazepine, an anticonvulsant with more efficacy for her bipolar issues rather than headaches; available as a longer-acting preparation, Oxtellar.
7. Angiotensin II receptor blockers (ARB)s such as candesartan (Atacand) or losartan. These would avoid the weight gain of the beta blockers. Candesartan has been the most studied of this group.
8. Muscle relaxants such as tizanidine, cyclobenzaprine, etc.

It should be noted in Heather's chart that lithium is a possibility, not for the headaches but for the bipolar issues. Lithium is underused, and many mildly bipolar patients state that they "finally feel normal" once lithium is given. In addition, the atypicals, such as quetiapine (Seroquel), or aripiprazole (Abilify) may be useful not only for Heather's moods but for the headaches as well.

Drugs that we want to avoid include the tricyclics (amitriptyline, nortriptyline, etc.), as they may exacerbate the bipolar illness and cause weight gain.

If Heather is on adequate mood-stabilizing medication, we may be able to utilize antidepressants. The use of antidepressants in bipolar patients is still controversial. For some, they help the depression with no side effects but, in others, even a small dose will trigger hypomania. If Heather is on mood stabilizers, we may be able to add a small dose of a selective serotonin reuptake inhibitor (SSRI) or similar med.

Beta blockers are also to be avoided, as we do not want to incur weight gain, and these may exacerbate Heather's depression. If a patient's headaches are improved but she gains 20 lbs and is always tired from the medicine, it is not the answer in the long run.

**What about other abortive possibilities?**

For other abortive possibilities, we would note in the chart the following:

Other triptans; if sumatriptan does not work out, it is worthwhile to use another triptan. Since these are far superior to our other choices, it is worthwhile to try at least three before giving up on the class.

Other NSAIDS (she is on naproxen); NSAIDS are not addicting and do not cause fatigue. Cambia is a powdered form of diclofenac potassium, and is Food and Drug Administration (FDA) indicated for migraine; NSAIDS may be combined with triptans.

Prodrin; this is a good combination of a mild vasoconstrictor, 20 mg caffeine, and acetaminophen. Prodrin fits the bill as a nonaddicting or sedating milder medicine and is useful for moderate headaches. We need to be careful with the amount of caffeine, however.

Dihydroergotamine (DHE) is primarily a venoconstrictor, not arterial, rendering it safer than other ergots.

We would also consider other antiemetic meds, such as prochlorperazine. We did prescribe ondansentron, one of the antiemetics that does not cause sedation.

## *Heather's Second Visit, 6 Weeks Later*

Heather reports that the topiramate has lessened the frequency of the migraines, and the daily headaches are not quite as severe. However, she is having a difficult time with her memory, and does not feel that she can increase the dose past 50 mg. The depression is possibly worse on the topiramate, but she wishes to continue with it, as it "is the first drug that has decreased the severity of my headaches."

Over-the-counter (OTC) naproxen helps her to some degree, and she is limiting her caffeine to 150 mg daily. For the migraines, the sumatriptan helps only 25 %, but the ondansentron is effective for her nausea.

Heather has begun to see a psychotherapist, who is teaching her to do biofeedback. She feels that this is helpful. She is exercising 20 min daily, on average.

**What would you consider as far as Heather's daily preventive meds at this time?**

We chose to continue with the topiramate, as it has helped. We cannot increase the dose, due to the cognitive side effects. Because of the depression, which is probably mild bipolar, we add quetiapine (Seroquel). It is important to begin with low doses of quetiapine, as many patients will quit the drug due to sedation. We start with 25 mg at night, and increase to 50 mg after 1 week. The atypicals carry the warning of an increased risk of developing diabetes and, of course, this must be communicated through informed consent. For most patients, I try to utilize as low a dose as is effective. Naturally, we warn Heather about possible sedation and weight gain. Some bipolar patients will have a paradoxical reaction to certain atypicals, and actually experience hypomania, usually mild. For the bipolar, lithium carbonate is a strong consideration.

**For Heather's abortives, the sumatriptan was only mildly effective; what would you consider?**

I do not want to quit the triptan class, as these are the most likely meds to stop the migraine, with minimal side effects. I would substitute rizatriptan, one tablet every 3 h prn, three in a day at most. The naproxen, limited to one or two OTC tabs per day, has been useful for her daily headaches, and ondansentron helps her nausea. She has only used three tabs of hydrocodone as an "escape" analgesic.

## *Summary*

Heather is currently on: topiramate, 50 mg qhs, quetiapine, slowly increasing to 50 mg qhs, and prn she uses OTC naproxen, rizatriptan, and ondansentron, with occasional hydrocodone as a backup.

In addition, Heather is watching triggers (regular meals, sleeping on time, etc.), exercising 20 min per day, and seeing a psychotherapist for therapy and biofeedback.

## *Two Weeks Later: A Call from Heather*

She reports that the quetiapine seems to help her mood the following day, but is sedating and she cannot take more than 25 mg at night. Rizatriptan has not been helpful and she had to resort to the hydrocodone for her last migraine.

**Would you change meds on the phone at this point and, if so, what would you consider?**

Since Heather seems to tolerate the low dose of quetiapine fairly well, and it may be starting to help her moods, we would continue this drug. On a mood stabilizer, such as lithium, lamotrigine, or quetiapine, Heather may be able to tolerate a low-dose antidepressant.

As far as her abortive medicines, the sumatriptan and rizatriptan have not been particularly effective. At this point, it is worthwhile to try one more triptan, either sumatriptan injections, the most effective form, or zolmitriptan (Zomig) nasal spray. Since she does not want to give herself an injection, we would prescribe the Zomig nasal spray. As usual, the instructions will be to use this early in the headache. This is a very effective triptan that partly bypasses the GI tract and has a relatively quick onset of action.

Note: All three sections of this case study are updated versions of articles that appeared in *Practical Pain Management* (PPM); this article was originally in *PPM,* Vol. 8, October 2008.

## An Interactive Case of Chronic Migraine: Part 2

*A step-by-step guide through the continued diagnosis and treatment of a refractory complex headache patient.*

Our patient Heather (not her real name) initially came in at age 24 and we chronicled her history and early treatment. In summary, Heather has moderate daily headache (chronic daily headaches, CDH), with migraine six times per month. She also suffers from anxiety and depression (the mild end of the bipolar spectrum). Heather has IBS (primarily diarrhea) plus neck pain. She was prescribed topiramate as a preventive with the following as abortives: sumatriptan, naproxen, ondansentron (for nausea), and occasional hydrocodone (see Appendix A for a complete list of generic/brand names of medications referred to in this chapter). Heather reports that the topiramate helped her headaches but possibly exacerbated her depression and caused mild memory disturbances. Fifty milligrams of topiramate is the most she can tolerate, as she experiences memory disturbances at a higher dose. Sumatriptan is only mildly helpful but OTC naproxen is useful and ondansentron relieves her nausea. She exercises 20 min daily, sees a therapist, and is learning biofeedback. We added quetiapine, slowly increasing to 50 mg at night, and substituted rizatriptan for sumatriptan. Quetiapine helps her moods but she cannot tolerate more than 25 mg qhs. Rizatriptan was not all that helpful, and during our last visit we prescribed zolmitriptan (Zomig) nasal spray.

Heather returned 6 months later at age 25. Her menstrual migraines are severe but zolmitriptan nasal spray helps (with naproxen) at least most of the time. Heather cycles in and out of depression, alternating with hypomania. She is chronically somewhat irritable and angry which interferes with relationships. Heather has had a rough go of it lately. She has a deadbeat boyfriend, Eric, who somehow neglected to inform her of his wife and two kids, and she also deals with an alcoholic, abusive mom (Sandy). Heather does not ruminate about suicide but occasionally wishes she were dead. She has no active suicidal plans. Heather loves her job, finds solace in the salon, but has been bickering with Alan, a new stylist who has been stealing some clients. So, along with headaches and neck pain, Heather is angry and depressed. She finds herself looking at every young, married woman with envy. Her two sisters are fairly supportive.

### *What Treatment Options Should Be Considered?*

Of course, we have a long talk with Heather about psychotherapy. She is reluctant to go, due to money, time, and stigma. We push Heather, suggesting a "sliding scale" therapist or a publicly funded therapy organization. We try to "destigmatize" going to therapy. I often say, "If it was up to me, everybody in our country would see a therapist." I have found that it may take many years of pushing and suggesting to convince reluctant patients to seek therapy.

Heather's headaches are somewhat controlled on 50 mg of topiramate and 25 mg of quetiapine with the following abortives: zolmitriptan nasal spray (Zomig), naproxen, ondansentron (for nausea), and occasional hydrocodone. Her moods are more of an issue at this point. We should search for medication options that may help Heather's (mild) bipolar moods as well as the headaches. Possibilities include: lamotrigine, oxcarbazepine, sodium valproate, another atypical (such as aripiprazole), or lithium. Ideally, we would like to avoid antidepressants, although some with bipolar who are on an adequate mood stabilizer may tolerate antidepressants. Lamotrigine would be the first choice as it has minimal side effects (rarely does lamotrigine cause tiredness or weight gain). Oxcarbazepine is a mild (and often overlooked) mood stabilizer. While related to carbamazepine, oxcarbazepine has markedly fewer adverse effects. There is a long-acting form of oxcarbazepine, Oxtellar. Sodium valproate may help moods as well as Heather's headaches. However, valproate does tend to cause weight gain and fatigue and greatly increases risks with pregnancy. Heather is on quetiapine but another atypical—such as aripiprazole—could help as it does not tend to cause the weight gain and fatigue that quetiapine may produce. Lithium in low doses is often very effective. Lithium is probably underutilized in the "mild" bipolar population. However, with lithium, particularly in higher doses, weight gain, fatigue, and hypothyroidism somewhat limit its use.

We decide to proceed with lamotrigine, slowly increasing to 100 mg daily. The risk with lamotrigine is Stevens–Johnson syndrome (SJS) as well as toxic epidermal necrolysis (TEN). These serious systemic and skin reactions are only observed in approximately 1 in 2500 patients to 3000 patients on lamotrigine. A "regular" drug rash is often seen (in at least 10 % of patients). With any rash, I stop the lamotrigine (or any drug new to the patient). SJS is an immunologically based, severe form of erythema multiforme. SJS and TEN are probably manifestations (SJS at the milder end of the spectrum, TEN more severe) of the same disease process. SJS usually involves the mucous membranes and skin. With SJS, the male-to-female ratio is 2:1 in patients with a genetic predisposition. Infectious SJS begins with nonspecific upper respiratory infection (URI) symptoms, with a sudden onset of skin lesions. Drug causes are varied—from oxicam NSAIDs to sulfa to anticonvulsants. The more severe TEN implies more skin area involvement than is seen with SJS. TEN carries a mortality rate of 30–50 % (while SJS has a mortality rate of 1–5 %).

We give Heather 25 mg of lamotrigine, to increase after 10 days to 50 mg. Some patients do well on low doses (25 mg), while others require 300 or 400 mg per day. Heather calls 3 weeks later and reports that she has not had a rash but has had no improvement in moods. We increase the lamotrigine to 75 mg for 10 days, then 100 mg per day. She is, of course, instructed to discontinue lamotrigine with any rash.

Six weeks later, Heather comes in and states that her mood is significantly improved. She is less irritated and depressed, and her mind racing is less. She has been working out her work differences with Alan, but the economy and decreased business helps fuel her depression. Mind racing may be a result of several conditions, particularly anxiety versus mania (or hypomania). It is important to inquire as to the "quality" of the rumination and racing. If it is constant worry, anxiety is the likely cause. With hypomania, it may simply be random thoughts racing through the brain and not necessarily connected to worry or anxiety.

Heather's headaches are more severe on the lamotrigine. She is now on 50 mg of topiramate as a headache preventive; 25 mg of quetiapine for moods, sleep, headache; and 100 mg of lamotrigine for moods (although lamotrigine may also alleviate headaches in some patients). It is possible that the lamotrigine has exacerbated Heather's headaches. This is a common situation with comorbid conditions where we are juggling various meds: A drug may help one condition while worsening another. At this point, Heather's moods are better on lamotrigine but headaches are more severe.

## *What Medication Changes Should Be Considered?*

We could add meds for Heather's headaches or decrease the lamotrigine. I usually choose to decrease medication that is causing significant side effects rather than add more medication. There are exceptions to this as, for instance, when a patient finally finds a drug that is the only one that has ever been helpful. With Heather, we choose to reduce the dose of lamotrigine from 100 to 75 mg/day. This may help her headache situation but, if not, we may need to decrease further. However, lamotrigine has been very helpful for Heather's moods and we will try to work with the drug.

At this point, Heather is 26 years old and on lamotrigine (75 mg), topiramate (50 mg), and quetiapine (25 mg). Due to side effects, she cannot tolerate more of any of these. Her moods and irritability improved on lamotrigine but headaches are not well controlled. Botulinum toxin type A (Botox) injections are now given to Heather, 16 units in each temple and frontal (totaling 48 units; this is considered a low dose). Botox is the only brand that has the FDA indication for chronic migraine. Botulinum toxin has a 55–65 % chance of producing reasonable improvement for 2–3 months. Some patients require 100–200 units. The official FDA indicated dose is 155 units, via 31 injections; other doses are considered to be "off-label." Repeated injections over time (every 3 months for 1 year) may have a beneficial, cumulative effect. Botulinum toxin (Botox) probably works at the neuronal level via anti-inflammatory mechanisms. Botulinum may be an effective inhibitor of the inflammatory compound, calcitonin gene-related peptide (CGRP), which is crucial in the propagation of CM pain.

Heather is now seeing a psychotherapist to deal with many issues. She has stopped seeing her terrible boyfriend and is learning to set limits with her difficult, alcoholic mom. Heather is doing yoga and exercising and is much more positive about her future. Massage has not been very helpful. She tried acupuncture, which can be beneficial, but her results were short-lived. We will next consider food sensitivity testing due to her migraines and IBS.

For 3 months post-botulinum injections, Heather's headaches are 40 % improved. We redo the low-dose (48 units) botulinum injections, which help her for 2.5 months. Her moods are improved and we leave the meds alone.

One year later, at age 27, Heather's headaches increase to a daily moderate migraine. Her moods remain stable on lamotrigine and quetiapine. We increase the topiramate, but 50 mg is the maximum she can tolerate. We are not sure if the topiramate is still helpful. This is commonly seen with preventive meds as they may lose effectiveness over time. The only way to evaluate if the med is still somewhat effective is to decrease or discontinue it. Many patients can only tolerate 25 or 50 mg of topiramate. She cannot afford botulinum toxin A injections, as her financial situation has taken a turn for the worse with the hair salon closing. Heather is also experiencing widespread pain with tenderness in many muscle groups. She saw a rheumatologist and was diagnosed as having fibromyalgia (FM). She now has three commonly linked "central sensitization" syndromes: migraine, IBS, and FM. It is common for central sensitization syndromes to be grouped together. The headaches and FM pain greatly affects her quality of life. Aside from medication, we encourage Heather to continue with exercise, yoga, and to take her vitamin D which may help depression and headaches, among other conditions. She tried acupuncture, but the relief lasted only 2 days.

## *What Other Medication Options Should Be Considered?*

Various medication choices include:

1. Adding a muscle relaxant,
2. Opioids (not a great choice at her young age of 27, it would be a last resort),
3. Short course of a low-dose steroid, which could exacerbate her bipolar and will only help for a brief period, or
4. Add an antidepressant used for pain, such as the tricyclics, duloxetine (Cymbalta), etc. She is on mood stabilizers, and may be able to tolerate low doses of an antidepressant without becoming hypomanic.

Heather has cycled back into a depression, primarily due to losing the salon job. She is lonely and under financial stress. We encourage Heather to get back into psychotherapy but she is reluctant to do so. Therapy is crucial for many reasons and, in Heather's situation, she has somewhat recreated her childhood abuse by being with an abusive man. Unfortunately, recreating childhood pathology as an adult is all too common. With the depression, Heather is no longer working out and has been overeating. She is back together with Eric, her lying, abusive boyfriend. Unfortunately, it is all too common for women to go back to an abusive relationship. Childhood pathological relationships (Heather has a very difficult mother) often are played out and repeated in adulthood and make the case for psychotherapy. Unfortunately, the reality is that most people with difficult childhoods do not receive the long-term therapy that is necessary to work through the attendant issues.

Because of the chronic pain (FM, headache) and depression, we add a low dose (30 mg) of duloxetine. Heather finds it is too stimulating and, while not hypomanic, she cannot sleep. We add a low dose (10 mg) of nortriptyline at night. Nortriptyline is a (milder) metabolite of amitriptyline with less sedation and anticholinergic side effects. Tricyclics such as these may be helpful for sleep, headache, FM, and IBS with diarrhea. Heather has all of these conditions. In an effort to minimize medication, we attempt to find drugs that treat several comorbidities simultaneously. Heather tolerates the nortriptyline well, with minimal sedation and dry mouth. Due to her bipolar, we may not be able to raise the dose of nortriptyline past 25 mg.

Six months later, at age 28, Heather is improved as far as moods and headache. She is working at a new salon, has left Eric (her terrible boyfriend) and is now in a group therapy. She exercises and continues to practice yoga.

## *Role of Genetic Resilience*

Despite her past abuse, Heather has shown some resilience. There is a major genetic component to resilience and that is the length of the serotonin transporter gene. In the face of childhood abuse (e.g., physical, sexual, emotional), it is predictable how an individual will function in adulthood by examining the shape of the serotonin gene. Two long arms to the gene are good, two short arms usually leads to a dysfunctional adult (with severe personality disorder pathology). Nature and nurture also comes into play. If a person has two short arms (bad) but a very good, nonabusive childhood, they usually will be ok. If one has two long arms to the gene (good), they usually are fairly functional and do well as adults—even in the face of abuse.

In a prospective monkey study, Bennet et al. [1] took two groups of very young monkeys with one group having the short-armed gene and the other having the long-armed gene. They then gave those monkeys an "abusive" childhood by having them raised not by mom but by the other adolescent monkeys. Those monkeys with the long arms to the gene did fairly well and showed normal functioning as adult monkeys. Those with short arms to the gene were dysfunctional, sitting in the corner, being asocial, biting, etc.

In our case history here, Heather had significant abuse as a child, but does not have a personality disorder and has shown resilience and insight, so she probably has two long arms to the gene. Unfortunately, abuse as a child influences the developing neurotransmitter pathways and often results in moderate or severe psychopathology, as well as chronic pain.

## *Conclusion*

We will revisit Heather at age 30 in a later article. She is on a common mix of mood stabilizers, antidepressants, and abortive meds. Botulinum toxin has been helpful.

While her history and medications are somewhat complex, I believe that situations similar to hers are commonly encountered in practice. Note: this is an updated version of an article that originally appeared in *PPM*, Vol. 10, October 2010.

## An Interactive Case History: Part 3

*A step-by-step guide through the continued diagnosis and treatment of a complex refractory headache patient.*

This is the third part of our series titled "Chronic Migraine: An Interactive Case History." Our previous articles [3, 4] followed the diagnosis of a complex patient with the pseudonym "Heather" from age 24 to 30. To recap, Heather has been suffering from migraine and CDH with neck pain. She has medical diagnoses of IBS and FM.

Heather's case is further complicated by chronic, mild bipolar depression and anxiety. She has been prescribed topiramate to prevent the migraines, which has helped but causes some side effects, including memory problems and paresthesias. Heather has also been taking a small dose, 25 mg, of quetiapine with the following abortive agents: 100 mg oral sumatriptan, zolmitriptan nasal spray, naproxen, ondansentron (for nausea), and hydrocodone in limited amounts. Botox injections were helpful but too expensive.

In addition to medications, Heather exercises, does yoga and biofeedback, and has seen a psychotherapist. Acupuncture and massage have not been useful.

### *History*

Heather is a 30-year-old hairdresser in a salon. Her work can be very physical, and her life has not been easy. She has an ex-boyfriend, Eric, who was abusive; she also was abused by her mom, Sandy, an alcoholic.

A few months ago, Heather ended her relationship with Eric. Now she is trying to turn her life around and is taking college classes at night. She has a new boyfriend, Steve, who is 15 years older and has two kids of his own. Heather is currently on 50 mg of topiramate and 25 mg of quetiapine to prevent headaches but cannot tolerate higher doses of either medication. Her irritability and anxiety have complicated her relationships with Steve and her coworkers at the hair salon. Heather is asking us: "Can you give me something else for my moods?"

## What Treatment Options Should Be Considered?

As noted, Heather's mood has been diagnosed on the mild end of the bipolar spectrum. When you suspect a patient may have a mood disorder, it is important to look for signs of a persistently agitated personality, with frequent cyclical depression or excessive energy, and a strong family history of either bipolar disorder or major depressive disorder. A family history of drug and/or alcohol abuse is also common. A clear hypomanic or manic episode may, however, not be evident. It is crucial to speak with a family member—at least 40 % of the time, hypomania is not mentioned or recognized when we simply speak with the patient.

Other mild bipolar signs include early onset of depression (teen years), quick onset of depression, severe depression "for no reason," opposite reactions to certain medications (such as being up all night with sedatives, mind racing from antidepressants, etc.), very high anxiety, insomnia, persistent agitation, a moody personality, and a poor response to antidepressants. Hypomania may manifest itself as a cycle of irritable, brooding pessimism. Depression is the primary problem, much more than the hypomania. Left untreated, self-medication is common.

Whereas an SSRI or serotonin–norepinephrine reuptake inhibitor (SNRI) may be the treatment of choice for Heather's mood disorder, these may trigger hypomania. In the past, lamotrigine increased her headaches but did help her mood significantly, whereas oxcarbazepine and sodium valproate gave her side effects.

We decide to add a small amount of an atypical antipsychotic, aripiprazole (Abilify), to Heather's regimen. Aripiprazole contains the same class warnings as the other atypical antipsychotics (primarily the risk for diabetes), but is much less apt to cause significant weight gain. With patients with headache who have psychiatric comorbidities, it is best to begin with low doses of medications. We usually begin with tiny doses (1/2 of a 2-mg tablet, slowly increasing to 5 or 10 mg). The common side effects associated with aripiprazole include akathisia, fatigue, headache, nausea, constipation, dizziness, insomnia, and visual disturbances.

Heather is begun on 1 mg of aripiprazole, increasing to 2 mg after 6 days. She is continued on her preventive regimen of 50 mg of topiramate and 25 of quetiapine. Oral sumatriptan has become ineffective for her migraines. Although the zolmitriptan nasal spray does help, it is no longer covered under her medical insurance. Financial considerations often dictate which medications we prescribe. The other generic triptan, naratriptan, is prescribed for Heather; she may use naratriptan with naproxen at the same time.

Six weeks later, Heather calls and states that she is pregnant.

## How does Pregnancy Affect Treatment?

Prior to her pregnancy, we had discussed the risks of taking headache medications with Heather. She and Steve had not planned on having a child right away. So, we now quickly taper her off the headache medications; whether to continue psychiatric medications during pregnancy is a difficult, case-by-case decision.

Our medication choices during pregnancy are limited. For headache treatment, acetaminophen is useful. The addition of caffeine may be beneficial. The triptans are pregnancy category C agents and therefore not often recommended during pregnancy. Although the sumatriptan pregnancy registry indicates that incidental use of sumatriptan during pregnancy may be relatively safe, we attempt to avoid its use during pregnancy. The risk of sumatriptan, as with most of our medications, is not definitively known. In addition to the 16 year sumatriptan/naratriptan study, a newer Norway study also indicates that triptans do not pose a major risk for birth defects. Of course, it is best to try and wait until after the first trimester prior to using a triptan.

In addition, we avoid barbiturate-containing drugs, such as butalbital. Prednisone, in very limited amounts, may be considered. Ondansentron, OTC Emetrol, and metoclopramide can be used for nausea during pregnancy.

For treatment of Heather's headaches, we prescribe ice, biofeedback/relaxation, acetaminophen with limited amounts of caffeine, minimal amounts of hydrocodone, and ondansentron for nausea.

As for preventives, propranolol, in limited amounts, has been used during pregnancy. Verapamil has also been used and has relatively fewer risks during pregnancy. Magnesium and omega-3 fatty acids may be used. Most medications, such as topiramate, are pregnancy category C agents, and the risks are not definitively known. Tricyclic antidepressants (TCAs) are best avoided. There is more leeway with these meds after the first trimester.

With regard to psychotropics, the atypical antipsychotics (quetiapine, aripiprazole, etc.) may turn out to be relatively safe, but definitive answers on these are still pending. There is a "neonatal SSRI syndrome," with the infant showing signs of jitteriness, increased muscle tone, irritability, and respiratory distress. Up to 30 % of infants exposed to SSRIs during the third trimester may have this syndrome.

With SSRIs, the issues of low birth weight, premature delivery, and neonatal pulmonary hypertension are possible complications, but studies have been conflicting. There have been other issues raised with SSRI use, such as an increased risk for attention deficit hyperactivity disorder (ADHD) and (possibly) autism in the child. Paroxetine is best avoided. Sertraline is the SSRI most often used and may be the safest SSRI during pregnancy. If possible, withdrawal off of the antidepressant should strongly be considered. Regarding mood stabilizers, lithium may be used but has some rare associated defects including Ebstein's anomaly, a cardiac valve defect. Valproate must be avoided. Lamotrigine is much safer than valproate but may cause cleft palate, among other problems. We usually avoid benzodiazepines. Buspirone (Buspar) is class B. As always, risks versus benefits and informed consent are important areas of discussion with the patient. For more information, refer to Organization of Teratology Information Services (OTIS) at otispregnancy.org or call 866-626-6847; also drugs.com (and similar sites).

Nerve blocks with lidocaine (class B) may be administered (particularly occipital blocks). For frontal pain, sphenopalatine ganglion (SPG) blocks with lidocaine are safe. The SPG blocks are usually done via the newer SphenoCath device, or the Tx360 unit. Of course, all treatment during pregnancy must be done with informed consent and with consideration of risk/benefit.

## *Stress at Home*

Heather's mother, Sandy, has been drinking more alcohol and "borrowing" money from Heather. Sandy is a continued source of stress, and she does not get along well with Steve, Heather's boyfriend. Heather's old therapist retired and she would like to see a new one, but money and time are barriers to seeing a therapist.

Heather calls and is very upset—she has had a miscarriage during week 8 of her pregnancy. Post miscarriage, Heather plunges into a deep depression. She has a reasonable support system consisting of Steve and her sister Emily. She is able to work at her salon. For the depression, we restart her medications (25 mg of quetiapine, 2 mg aripiprazole). For the headache and FM pain, we again add 10 mg of nortriptyline at night. Heather did reasonably well on nortriptyline in the past, without hypomania. For crisis times, with both headache and depression, I often retreat back to medications that have been helpful in the past. Some bipolar patients tolerate antidepressants well, without hypomania, particularly if they are on a mood stabilizer. Others become manic or hypomanic. It is important to begin with low doses of an antidepressant and increase the amount slowly.

## *At this Point, Would you Consider Botulinum Toxin or Occipital Nerve Blocks?*

Heather has insurance coverage again and requests that we administer botulinum toxin type A (Botox). Botox is FDA approved for the treatment of CM (defined as 15 days per month, 4+ h per day of migrainous headache). The FDA-indicated protocol is 31 injections at various sites about the head and neck; 155 total units. I often use lower doses, from 50 to 100 botox units per patient. We give Heather 75 total units (15 injections, 5 units each), injected into the anterior as well as posterior areas.

Because she has been suffering from severe daily migraine with occipital pain and tenderness, we also administer occipital blocks with bupivacaine. Although the addition of corticosteroid in the occipital injection may help, I usually avoid adding steroids. Occipital injections often help until the botox injections are effective, which may take 1–4 weeks. Frontally, SPG blocks are a consideration.

Now aged 32, Heather is seeing a new psychotherapist. She is encouraged to join Al-Anon to deal with her mom's drinking. Heather has dropped out of community college because of her depression. She has been able to continue working but is under-functioning at work. Both headaches and depression are major contributors to this. Heather's boyfriend, Steve, has recently begun using cocaine again, and Heather joins in. The cocaine cycles Heather into hypomania.

## *What Treatment Should Be Considered?*

In the past, Heather has been referred to psychiatrists and psychotherapists. She is willing to see a therapist, but not a psychiatrist, as she says, "It never works out with any psychiatrist. I do not connect and it is too expensive." Steve recently went into rehab, but Heather rejects the idea of rehab. With the help of a therapist, she is able to quit cocaine on her own, which is unusual.

We increase the aripiprazole to 5 mg and reintroduce lamotrigine. Heather is now on quetiapine (25 mg at night), aripiprazole (5 mg every morning), and lamotrigine (25 mg, slowly increasing to 100 mg). We have warned Heather to discontinue lamotrigine with any sign of a rash. The Botox has decreased her headaches for 3 months, but she can no longer afford the injections.

Steve breaks up with Heather after he finishes rehab for cocaine. Heather moves in with her supportive sister, Emily, which stabilizes her situation. Heather does reasonably well, working at her salon, for more than 2 years. At age 33, she continues to work on a number of issues with her therapist, including her difficult mom.

Heather begins to date Eric again. The relationship is stable for 6 months, after which he begins, once again, to abuse her. Heather cannot afford aripiprazole and is on quetiapine and lamotrigine. As needed, she uses naratriptan and ondansentron, but we do not give her hydrocodone because of her bout with cocaine. She is at high risk for addiction because of her bipolar disorder, alcoholic mom, cocaine use, and stressful life. We periodically do occipital blocks and trigger point injections, but she cannot afford Botox. Heather now admits that she is ingesting six Extra Strength Excedrin daily, along with eight ibuprofen. She has severe GI pain as a result.

## *Weaning off OTC Pain Medications*

Medication overuse is common among chronic daily headache patients; it is almost a part of the illness. Some patients, maybe most patients, will have medication overuse headache, whereas other patients who overuse analgesics do not suffer from rebound headache. Treating patients with medication overuse is difficult; the brain becomes "centrally sensitized," and patients are psychologically and physically dependent on the analgesics. There are a number of protocols for weaning off the various analgesics.

We place Heather on a proton-pump inhibitor (PPI; omeprazole) to treat her GI issues. She agrees to stop taking the OTC Excedrin and ibuprofen and switch to a nonaddicting muscle relaxant, tizanidine. Heather is tapered off caffeine over 3–5 weeks; overuse of caffeine is a major problem in headache patients. Of course, patients are not always truthful about their OTC and caffeine use. We order blood work; in headache patients, routine blood laboratories are vital because of the medications prescribed (and overuse). Heather's liver is mildly irritated, which we would expect to improve over time as long as she is off the analgesics. We restart nortriptyline 10 mg at night and increase lamotrigine to 150 mg, which helps her moods. However, with the increase in the lamotrigine, Heather's headaches increase. We decrease the dose of the lamotrigine to 100 mg.

Because of her abusive relationship with Eric, Heather moves to a woman's shelter and is temporarily lost to follow up. When she returns for therapy 8 months later, she is off all medications, unemployed, and very depressed. We place her back on 25 mg of topiramate and 25 mg of quetiapine, with naratriptan and ondansentron as needed.

The new regimen stabilizes Heather's condition, and she is able to live with her sister Emily and go back to working at the salon. She improves psychologically and finds a new therapist. Her mother, Sandy, who is living with Heather and Emily, is a continuing source of stress. The therapist has convinced Heather to enforce boundaries with her mother. Heather is exercising and doing yoga. She tries the herbal preventive Petadolex, the most effective "natural" headache preventive, but it does not help. Magnesium oxide or citrate is the second most effective "natural" preventive.

## *Conclusion*

Heather is now 35 years old. She reunites with her older boyfriend, Steve, and they become engaged. She wants to become pregnant, and we discuss risks and benefits of the various medications.

Heather decides to continue on the mood stabilizer quetiapine for the time being. She is able to take a small amount (5 mg) of cyclobenzaprine, which helps her FM and insomnia. She feels somewhat "drugged" in the morning because of the muscle relaxant. We use flurbiprofen, an NSAID, 100 mg once or twice daily. We give Heather Prodrin to use no more than twice per day. Prodrin (acetaminophen, caffeine, and isometheptene) is an improved and nonsedating form of Midrin (Epidrin). Naratriptan helps her, but she tends to overuse the triptans, consuming up to 27 per month. Limiting the analgesics is a continuing battle with Heather, as with many daily headache sufferers. Heather's moods are relatively stable for the moment, and she continues to plan for a baby.

## Appendix A
## Generic and Brand Names of Drugs Cited in this Article

| Generic | Brand |
|---|---|
| Amitriptyline | Elavil® |
| Aripiprazole | Abilify® |
| Botulinum toxin type A | Botox®, Dysport® |
| Carbamazepine | Tegretol® |
| Cortisone | Prednisone, Decadron, Medrol |
| Cyclobenzaprine | Flexeril |
| Duloxetine | Cymbalta® |
| Flurbiprofen | Ansaid |
| Hydrocodone | Vicodin®, Norco® |
| Lamotrigine | Lamictal® |
| Metoclopramide | Reglan |
| Naproxen | Naprosyn® |
| Naratriptan | Amerge |
| Nortriptyline | Pamelor® |
| Omeprazole | Prilosec |
| Ondansentron | Zofran® |
| Oxcarbazepine | Trileptal®, Oxtellar |
| Paroxetine | Paxil |
| Quetiapine | Seroquel® |
| Rizatriptan | Maxalt® |
| Sertraline | Zoloft |
| Sodium valproate | Depakote® |
| Sumatriptan | Imitrex® |
| Tizanidine | Zanaflex |
| Topiramate, topiramate ER | Topamax®, Trokendi XR |
| Verapamil | Calan, Isoptin |
| Zolmitriptan | Zomig® |

Petadolex is a form of the herb butterbur
Prodrin is a combination of acetaminophen, caffeine, and isometheptene
Note: This is an updated version of an article that originally appeared in *Practical Pain Management,* Vol. 11, April 2011

## Suggested Reading

1. Bennett AJ, Lesch KP, Heils A, Long JC, Lorenz JG, Shoaf SE, Champoux M, Suomi SJ, Linnoila MV, Higley JD (2002) Early experience and serotonin transporter gene variation interact to influence primate CNS function. Mol Psychiatry 7(1):118–122
2. Robbins L (2008a) Chronic migraine: an interactive case history. Pract Pain Manag 8(8):56–58
3. Robbins L (2008b) Chronic Migraine: an interactive case history: a step by step guide through the diagnosis of a complex headache patient. Pract Pain Manag 8(8):56–58
4. Robbins L, Snediker D (2010) Chronic migraine: an interactive case history, part 2. Pract Pain Manag 10(8):72–74

# Chapter 7
# Miscellaneous

## Case Studies in NDPH: New Daily Persistent Headache

**Case History #1, Adult** Jack is a 42-year-old male, with no prior history of headaches or migraines, and is in good overall health. Two years ago, he awoke with a mild headache, which became severe as the day progressed. He had been experiencing cold type symptoms for about a week, had been under severe stress, and was not sleeping well. Jack now suffers from a moderate daily headache that is continuous, 24/7.

A workup by his general practitioner (GP) was completely normal. He visited a succession of doctors: his chiropractor, acupuncturist, physical therapist, dentist, and psychotherapist, all to no avail. He was prescribed various analgesics and headache preventives over the next 2 years, but found nothing that helped. After 2 years, a neurologist diagnosed Jack with new daily persistent headache (NDPH). Jack has lost his job due to the head pain, and his marriage is suffering. The next step is to try onabotulinumtoxinA (Botox) injections.

**Case History #2, Adolescent** Rose is a 17-year-old female with no history of headaches. She presented with a severe headache that began suddenly 3 months prior, during finals of her junior year. A perfectionist, Rose is a straight A student who puts enormous pressure on herself. Rose has moderate anxiety, but no depression. She has a history of irritable bowel syndrome (IBS) that worsens under stress. Prior to visiting a headache specialist, she had not had a recent workup, nor had she seen an ophthalmologist. Her continuous headaches have interfered with school, and she is now homebound.

Her workup, consisting of laboratories, magnetic resonance imaging (MRI), and an ophthalmological exam, was normal. Topiramate was titrated to 150 mg, but it did not help, and produced intolerable side effects. Amitriptyline did help, but Rose gained weight and was very tired. Various abortives were utilized, but none was particularly helpful. A psychologist trained Rose in biofeedback, which was somewhat helpful for her head pain and IBS. Botox injections are being considered.

 
L. Robbins, *Advanced Headache Therapy*, DOI 10.1007/978-3-319-13899-2_7

## *Introduction*

New daily persistent headache (NDPH) is one type of chronic daily headache, along with chronic migraine, chronic tension headache, and hemicrania continua. NDPH is being increasingly recognized as an important type of headache, both because of the frequency and also the refractory nature of the head pain.

## *Onset and Symptoms*

NDPH develops quickly, usually within hours or 1 day, but within 3 days the headache must be constant [39]. Many patients remember exactly what they were doing when the headaches began. The pain is usually bilateral, with aching pressure and/or throbbing. The intensity may vary from mild to severe, but tends to be mild to moderate. The headache is usually constant. At least half of patients describe migraine-associated features, such as nausea, phonophobia, lightheadedness, photophobia, etc. Allodynia, often seen in chronic migraine, is present in approximately a quarter of patients [37]. Autonomic symptoms (nasal stuffiness, conjunctival injection, etc.) may occur.

## *Diagnosis*

NDPH is somewhat a diagnosis of exclusion. Infection (including meningitis and sinusitis), mass lesions, subdural hematomas, cerebral venous thrombosis, low or high cerebrospinal fluid (CSF) pressure headaches, arteritis, arterial dissection, posttraumatic, etc., all need to be excluded [10]. Usually the history, along with MRI/magnetic resonance angiogram (MRA), will exclude these entities. There are several newer proposed diagnostic classifications; generally, diagnosis includes:

- At least 3 months of sudden-onset headache
- No significant remission
- Exclusion of other disorders [14]

NDPH is unilateral in a small number of patients, and if this occurs with autonomic symptoms, it may represent a variant of hemicrania continua.

## *Pathophysiology*

While we do not know the pathophysiology of NDPH, central nervous system (CNS) inflammation is one possibility. Tumor necrosis factor-α (TNF-α) has been implicated in neuro-inflammation. TNF-α is a cytokine that enhances inflammation. In one study, CSF evaluations of NDPH patients resulted in almost all samples showing an increase in CSF TNF-α [40].

Glial cell disruption may play a role; glial cells manufacture CNS cytokines. Glial cells are very sensitive to viral infection and stress; surgery may impact glials as well [11]. Cervical joint hypermobility, along with hypermobility of other joints, may play a role [42]. Patients with NDPH often are tall and thin, with long necks.

## *Epidemiology*

CDH occurs in approximately 3.5 % of the population, but the prevalence of NDPH is not known. One study from a headache center concluded that 10.8 % of 638 CDH patients had NDPH [8]. A similar study in the pediatric population revealed that, among those with CDH, 13 % had NDPH [19]. NDPH may well be more prevalent among adolescents than in adults. Females outnumber males with NDPH by approximately 2.5 to 1 [10]. Most patients do not have a previous history of headache. A prior history of anxiety or depression is seen in about half of the NDPH patients [10]. After the onset of NDPH, many patients experience depression.

## *Triggering Events*

Approximately, 50 % of patients have an identifiable trigger. Stress may be a trigger in some patients. Infection, particularly viral, is often cited as a trigger [39]. In one study, the Epstein–Barr virus was implicated as an initiating culprit [7]. Exposure to certain toxins may also precede the onset of NDPH. Surgical procedures have occasionally triggered the onset of NDPH. Head injury, even when mild, may be an initial event. Cervical trauma or other pathology, particularly in those who have thin necks with cervical hypermobility, may initiate the onset of NDPH.

## *Treatment*

NDPH is more resistant to treatment than is chronic migraine, which is usually transformed migraine (slow onset over years). The usual daily preventive migraine medications are given, as they may be helpful for some NDPH patients. These include tricyclic antidepressants (amitriptyline, protriptyline, etc.), anticonvulsants (valproate, topiramate, etc.), antihypertensives (β-blockers, calcium channel blockers, etc.), Petadolex (natural butterbur), SSRIs (fluoxetine, sertraline, etc.), SNRIs (duloxetine, venlafaxine, etc.), and muscle relaxants (tizanidine, etc.). OnabotulinumtoxinA (Botox) may be helpful as well; there are no published controlled trials of treatment for NDPH. Benzodiazepines, particularly clonazepam, have had some limited success. Intravenous dihydroergotamine (IV DHE) is more likely to be of help with chronic migraine. A course of high-dose IV corticosteroids, followed by oral steroids, has shown some promise, but the high doses can predispose to serious side effects [36]. IV magnesium may provide short-term relief. Doxycycline, given over several months, may help some patients with NDPH. Greater occipital nerve blocks sometimes are useful, particularly with unilateral headaches. Sphenopalatineganglion (SPG) frontal blocks, with the newer devices SphenoCath, Allevio, or Tx360, may help.

Outside of medication, psychotherapy is worthwhile for those with anxiety or depression. Biofeedback is helpful for some headache patients. Exercise is always encouraged, as is yoga and Pilates. Acupuncture, physical therapy, or chiropractic may help for some patients.

While the results of treatment may be discouraging, it is crucial to stick with the patient, continue to try different medications or modalities, and not to give up on the NDPH sufferer.

### *Long-Term Prognosis*

Several studies have evaluated long-term outcomes. One study revealed that, after 2 years with NDPH, about 25 % of the patients were free of headache, and 66 % had at least a 50 % reduction in pain levels [33]. Another study reported that 76 % of patients continued to have headaches over time, while 15 % remitted; median time to remission was 21 months. Eight percent had a cyclic form, with a relapsing-remitting pattern. A small study of children and adolescents discovered that 8 out of 28 patients were free of headache within 1–2 years, while most (20) continued to suffer long-term from head pain [53].

### *Conclusion*

NDPH is an important category of headache, as it is often difficult to treat, and results in considerable disability. It is unique in that more than 50 % of patients have an identifiable trigger, although these range from infection to surgery to head trauma. We are just beginning to identify the pathophysiology that leads to NDPH. Treatment of NDPH is scattershot and varied at present; further studies will undoubtedly lead to more effective therapies. Note this is a version of an article that originally was published in *Practical Pain Management*, Vol. 12, July 2012.

## The Immune System and Headache

*This chapter finds that the immune system plays a key role in migraine pathogenesis and that manipulation of immune system elements may be a promising area of development for new headache therapies.*

The involvement of the immune system in chronic headache has been speculated upon since the 1970s [47, 48]. Various components of the immune system have been examined in relation to headache [13, 25]. While great strides have been made in advancing our understanding of neuroimmunology, the complexities of the system make its specific role in headache pathology unclear. This chapter describes some of the key elements in the immune system and their relation to headache pathogenesis.

## *Calcitonin Gene-Related Peptide*

Calcitonin gene-related peptide (CGRP) in an inflammatory neuropeptide involved at every level of migraine pathophysiology, including the meninges, trigeminal ganglion, trigeminocervical complex, brain stem nuclei, thalamus, and the cortex. Upon initiation of migraine at the brain stem or cortex level, neurogenic inflammation occurs such that peripheral trigeminocervical neurons are activated. We then observe a release of CGRP and other neuroinflammatory peptides. CGRP induces neurogenic vasodilation that leads to further plasma protein extravasation (PPE) and the influx of mast cells and other pro-inflammatory cells [21]. The process of neurogenic inflammation sensitizes the peripheral nociceptors transmitting via the trigeminal axon, through the brain stem and the thalamus, and finally into the cortex.

In animal models, CGRP is released following stimulation of the CNS—similar to what is observed in migraine. Triptans inhibit the animal's CGRP release. In humans, injections of CGRP into migraine patients result in delayed headache. Certain studies have suggested that relief of migraine corresponds to a reduction of CGRP levels in the blood and that migraine-specific therapy with triptans decreases CGRP [45]. These studies have led to the development of CGRP-receptor antagonists that could conceivably block neurogenic vasodilation in the meninges. CGRP activity in the trigeminal ganglion may limit vasoconstriction.

Two CGRP-receptor antagonists, olcegepant and telcagepant, were tested for the abortive treatment of migraine; unfortunately, their development is on hold [22]. There are ongoing studies of monoclonal antibody injections, once per month, for the prevention of migraine.

It is possible that onabotulinumtoxin type A (Botox) may work via anti-inflammatory neuroimmune mechanisms. The effect of Botox may partially be due to its effect on CGRP, or other similar inflammatory compounds.

## *Cytokines*

Recent studies have revealed that the neuropeptide CGRP triggers the secretion of cytokines via stimulation of CGRP receptors found on T cells [5, 23]. Cytokines are involved in inflammation, in modulation of the pain threshold, and also in trigeminal nerve fiber sensitization. In small trials, cytokines have been proven to precipitate headache [51].

In trials where TNF was injected, headaches were shown to be induced while, on the other hand, the TNF antibody was shown to reduce pain in humans [54]. Plasma levels of both pro- and anti-inflammatory cytokines are enhanced during migraine attacks. TNF levels increase after migraine pain onset and decrease progressively over time after the onset of the attack [34]. Plasma levels of a pro-inflammatory cytokine, interleukin (IL)-1, are also enhanced after the initiation of headache. IL-1 release is induced by TNF and may lead to hyperalgesia. The amount of an anti-inflammatory cytokine, IL-10, has also been shown to increase after the onset of a headache and may be involved in analgesia. One study revealed IL-10 inhibited release of TNF, which is antinociceptive [49].

Cytokine levels in the CSF of migraineurs have been studied with varied results. Increases in IL-1 receptor antagonist (IL-1ra), monocyte chemoattractant protein-1 (MCP-1) and transforming growth factor-1 (TGF-1) were measured in patients with migraine and episodic tension-type headache (TTH) versus pain-free controls. Rather than being the cause of headache, changes in the level of cytokines in the CSF are thought to be due to pain [4]. No correlation has linked increased cytokine levels to a decrease in pain and there has not been a difference found in cytokine levels with migraine versus episodic TTH [4].

## *Tumor Necrosis Factor*

TNF is a pro-inflammatory cytokine involved in inflammation and it is crucial in the activation of pain. A small number of patients with NDPH develop symptoms after viral infection. It is possible that a pro-inflammatory cytokine such as TNF could initiate and maintain CNS inflammation even after the infection resolves. Rozen et al. [41] reported elevated levels of CSF TNF in 19 of 20 NDPH patients, in 16 of 16 chronic migraine patients, and in 2 of 2 chronic tension headache patients. The study suggests that TNF plays a role in the etiology of these types of headache. Refractory chronic daily headache could involve increased levels of CSF TNF. Patients with NDPH (and, theoretically, elevated TNF) often are refractory to a variety of medication regimens.

TNF is important in a number of conditions such as sinusitis and rhinitis, as well as headache [6]. The development of drugs that modulate TNF may prove beneficial to these conditions as well as headache.

## *Adiponectin*

Obesity is a known to be a major risk factor for the development of chronic migraine [35]. Adipose tissue secretes adipocytokine adiponectin, which is believed to modulate several inflammatory mediators important in migraine. A large amount of adipose tissue leads to decreased secretion of adiponectin [16]. Adiponectin has a protective role in limiting the development of insulin resistance, dyslipidemia, and atherosclerosis. It also has an anti-inflammatory action through inhibition of cytokines IL-6 and TNF-induced IL-8 production. Adiponectin induces the production of cytokine IL-10, which is anti-inflammatory. Adiponectin decreases migraine but, paradoxically, a sudden increase may worsen a headache [35].

## *Glia and Headache*

Recent studies have shown that glial cells, previously thought to serve only a supportive role, are now known to directly influence the microenvironment of trigeminal ganglion neurons through gap junctions and paracrine signaling [46]. Following trigeminal activation, CGRP secreted from neuronal cell bodies activates adjacent glial cells to release nitric oxide (NO) and inflammatory cytokines which, in turn, initiate inflammatory events in the trigeminal ganglia that lead to peripheral sensitization [6, 26]. The neuronal glial signaling is thought to be an important process, ultimately leading to the initiation of migraine. The glial modulation of neurons through immune mediators is an unexplored area for new migraine medications. An excellent report on glia research by Drs. Moskovitz and Cooper appeared in these pages in the November/December 2010 issue [31].

## *Mast Cells*

It is generally accepted that migraines are partially mediated by prolonged activation of meningeal nociceptors (pain receptors). One possible explanation of how this occurs seems to be found in the physiology of mast cells. Mast cells are granulated immune cells that play a critical role in inflammation. They have been found to reside in high density in the intercranial dura, a peripheral tissue covering the brain [8]. Mast cells are located in close proximity to the blood vessels and the primary afferent nociceptive neurons.

When the mast cells are stimulated, they degranulate their contents into the local milieu. This activates the surrounding trigeminal meningeal nociceptors and promotes a prolonged state of excitation. It is not clear if there is a specific molecule released from the mast cells that is responsible for the propagation of migraine. Several of the degranulated molecules have implications for migraine. The list includes histamine, leukotrienes, the cytokines TNF and IL-6, and endothelin-1 [43, 15].

Once the meningeal nociceptors are activated by the release of mast cell molecules, they propagate a cascade of neuronal activation by releasing neuropeptides (e.g., CGRP, substance P). These activate and further degranulate residual mast cells and thus prolong the migraine headache. According to Levy et al. [24], the key lies in the increased expression of the phosphorylated form of the extracellular signal-related kinase (pERK). This is an anatomical marker for nociceptor activation and downstream signaling of the spinal trigeminal nucleus.

## *Seasonal Allergies and Headache*

The association between seasonal allergies and headaches has been well documented in several studies [9, 1, 30, 52, 32, 29]. A recent study found that headaches are 1.5 times more common in those with atopic conditions (asthma, seasonal allergic rhinosinusitis, chronic bronchitis) than those without these disorders [1]. This relationship suggests that inflammatory changes in the nasal and sinus mucosa of individuals with seasonal allergic rhinosinusitis could be a potential trigger for migraines. Allergies may also partly explain the seasonal variation experienced by many migraine sufferers. However, several primary headache disorders, including migraine, are at least partly characterized by the presence of cranial autonomic symptoms (e.g., conjunctival injection, lacrimation, eyelid edema, rhinorrhea, nasal congestion, postnasal drip, and reddening of the face and ears) which closely resemble the signs and symptoms of seasonal allergic rhinosinusitis [9]. This overlap in symptomatic presentation can make it quite difficult to clinically distinguish headache secondary to seasonal allergic rhinosinusitis from primary headache associated with cranial autonomic symptoms. Accurate characterization of these headaches through a detailed history and physical examination is crucial since appropriate treatment highly depends upon a proper diagnosis.

Many patients who believe they have sinus headaches are suffering from migraine. In fact, sinus headache is the most common misdiagnosis of patients with migraine [9, 28, 3, 35]. For its part, the International Headache Society (IHS) does not recognize sinus headache as a diagnostic entity—unless it is associated with a confirmed diagnosis of underlying acute rhinosinusitis.

## *Conclusion*

The immune system plays a key role in migraine pathogenesis. The involvement of CGRP is important in neurogenic vasodilation, peripheral sensitization, and the initiation of the migraine cascade. Various cytokines, including TNF, IL-1, and adiponectin, have been implicated in the precipitation of migraine.

The role of allergies in migraine remains a confusing area. In headache-prone individuals, seasonal allergies may be a trigger and most people diagnosed with sinus headaches are actually suffering from migraine.

The earliest work on the immune system and headache focused on mast cells and their role in propagating the cascade of neuronal activation when degranulated. The supporting glia cells, long thought to be inert, have been found to modulate neuronal activity—partly through immune mediators. The manipulation of immune system elements is a promising area of development for new headache therapies, although these may be many years in development. Note this originally appeared in *Practical Pain Management*, Vol. 11, Jan 2011.

## Weight Loss

Weight loss and exercise may help headaches. Develop a long-term approach.

Different approaches work for different people. Permanent weight loss is difficult. It takes changes in lifestyle and behavior. It never comes about through wishfully thinking, "I need to lose a few pounds and exercise." It comes about via a concerted effort in which exercise and weight control become an important project in your life. You need to get up every morning committed to your program, focusing on how to get your needed exercise and sticking to your diet.

Key steps to maintaining a weight loss are:

- Grazing (eating small meals throughout the day while reducing portions at mealtime).
- Portion control (measure or weigh your food) *Portion control is crucial!* You cannot exercise off bad nutrition!
- Count calories or points. (Weight Watchers is a good program, as is the www.sparkpeople.com website.)
- Weigh yourself often.
- Eat foods that are low in fat, sugar and salt, and high in fiber.
- Do *not* diet. Severely restricting food is related to the yo-yo syndrome, where weight is frequently lost but quickly regained. When you fall off the wagon, get right back on your diet/exercise program; it is crucial to *not* let bad days turn into weeks and months. Diets do not work.
- Motivation is a key; dietitians/nutritionists can help. Fitness/health magazines are motivating. One good newsletter is the Nutrition Action Newsletter (www.cspinet.org). Apps such as myfitnesspal are helpful.
- The old Weight Watchers motto to "Move more and eat less" is still relevant. The Weight Watchers app is excellent.
- Exercise regularly; it has to be "fun"; people who view it as "exercise" eat more afterward
- The "turtle" wins the weight loss race.
- Try a "Fitbit" step counter (or other similar type).

Weight loss supplements (over the counter) do not work. For a review of these, and natural products, www.consumerlab.com is an excellent site. Medicines that may help weight loss:

1. Topiramate (one of the main migraine preventives): decreases appetite.
2. Stimulants: phentermine (and others) help: these are best used short term.

## Exercise: Just do Something and Have Fun!!

Exercising may decrease headaches. It is certainly crucial for weight loss. To get most of the benefits of exercise, you only need to think of exercising in small chunks of time, even 10 or 15 min. Most people are able to fit exercise more easily into their lives when thinking this way. We are looking for a total of 20 min daily on average. The more the merrier. Some people do well counting total minutes of exercise from Monday to Sunday, including everything (walking, etc.). Used fitness equipment places have good, inexpensive bikes.

It helps to have a routine, whether it is regular walks, classes, or equipment to use at home. A stationary bike is easy to use; you can read or watch TV while riding, and even 5 or 10 min at a time will add up. Studies have shown that short intervals of exercise throughout the day can be as effective as doing one prolonged session. I think that the old mantra of "getting your heart rate up to a target #, for an intense hour" actually kept people from exercising; the idea is to just do something, anything, for any period of time.

If you do not enjoy what you are doing, you will not continue it. Health clubs are great, and the classes are motivating. Pilates is core work, and is crucial for preventing back pain, and falls, as we age. There are DVD and Cable TV Pilates, but live classes are best. Five or ten minutes of Pilates or core work, three or four times per week, helps quite a bit. Yoga is also very good, and can help with stress and headaches. Even 5 or 10 min of yoga posing are beneficial. Consider using a personal trainer.

Remaining active throughout the day is also important. People who are moving throughout the day instead of sitting are in better shape than those who sit all day and exercise only at night. Standing at the computer may help the core, and taking frequent breaks from sitting is important. The Fitbit (or similar step counters) are motivating and helpful.

Many people get into diet and exercise, for a period of time, and then out of it. Getting back into exercise takes some inertia, such as just walking (or a stationary bike) for 5 min. Just do something for a few days, and you will get back "into it." Do not worry about "going to the club and getting my heart rate up and exercising hard for an hour." Just dive back in with baby steps.

## Supplements for Good Health (in Headache Patients)

*Vitamin D is important to take; everything else is very iffy*

Most herbal and vitamin supplements have not held up to scrutiny in controlled trials, and some have turned out to be harmful. A number of well-done studies have linked multivitamins and antioxidants (the supplements) to an increase in cancer, among other problems. Do not believe the advertising claims: Multivitamins and many other supplements are not necessary for good health, and could be harmful. www.consumerlab.com/ is an excellent site for info on vitamins and herbs. Even omega-3 capsules are now implicated in causing cancer. Antioxidants, particularly

A, C, and E, have been linked to high rates of cancer. Vitamin B and C can actually give you headaches. The only vitamin truly holding up to scrutiny is Vitamin D.

*Vitamin D* is important for our skin and bones, and may help fight hypertension and autoimmune diseases. Recently, adequate levels of vitamin D have been linked to lowered rates of cancer, especially colorectal cancer. People who live in cold climates are often low in vitamin D, as they are not in the sun enough. Most need to take a vitamin D supplement. The latest studies suggest that adults need at least 2000 international units a day. Avoid the generic vitamin D; use a name brand. The *Nature Made* brand available everywhere is US Pharmacopeia (USP)-certified and is an excellent brand. If you take calcium with added D, you probably still need to take an extra D supplement. Do not take more than 4000 units of vitamin D without consulting your physician.

**Omega-3s (Fatty Acids)** Many studies have shown the benefits of omega-3s (natural, not capsules) for the heart, for moods, and possibly for headaches. Eating fish twice a week is a good goal, particularly fatty fish such as salmon, tuna, trout, and mackerel. Other sources of omega-3s in the diet are tofu, soybeans, walnuts, and canola oil. It is better to get omega-3s naturally than from supplements. In fact, the supplements have been linked to increased cancer rates. We do not recommend the omega-3 supplements!

*Calcium* is necessary for the heart, muscles, and nerves to function and for blood to clot. Low intake of calcium leads to the development of osteoporosis and is associated with high rates of bone fractures. Absorption of calcium decreases as we age. Eating too much salt and protein, especially animal protein, increases calcium loss. It is much better to get calcium in foods than in supplements. Calcium supplements have had side effects, and should be taken only if you cannot get enough calcium in foods.

Calcium is found in milk, yogurt, cheese, broccoli, tofu, beans, sardines, calcium-enriched fruit juices, fortified cereals, etc. Our systems cannot absorb more than 500 mg of calcium at a time. Calcium in the form of calcium citrate, such as citracal, is more easily absorbed than calcium carbonate. Citracal caplets plus D are a good form of calcium (315 mg) plus vitamin D (200 IU). The usual dose is one or two tablets, once or twice a day; consult your physician. To learn more about calcium, visit www.health.nih.gov.

**Aspirin** If you are at risk for heart disease, your doctor may recommend a daily dose of aspirin. Its properties may help prevent heart attacks, strokes, and even headaches and certain cancers. The usual dose is one aspirin (325 mg) a day.

Generic aspirin is fine. Taking a baby aspirin (81 mg) or a half-tablet of regular aspirin (162 mg) may be sufficient; the dose varies by person. Aspirin can cause stomach ulcers; if it hurts your stomach or causes heartburn, stop taking it and consult your doctor.

*Coenzyme Q10 (CoQ10)*, for people on statins, is a crucial compound, important for your heart, muscles, and nerves. It is naturally produced by your body. However, the statins (cholesterol-lowering drugs like Simvastatin, Lipitor, Pravachol, Vytorin, and Crestor) deplete the body's CoQ10.

Studies have indicated a possible benefit from CoQ10 for migraine and the heart. We suggest taking 200 mg per day of CoQ10 if you take one of the statin drugs. It has not yet been proven that this helps the muscles, but CoQ10 is generally safe and may prevent headaches.

**Resources** An excellent newsletter, Nutrition Action Health Letter, is inexpensive (Visit www.cspinet.org). A good website for healthy living is www.sparkpeople.com, with more than a million members. We also like www.consumerlab.com.

## Chaos (Nonlinear Dynamics) and Migraine

*Note: This article is included primarily for interest sake, and also because chaotic mechanisms may be important in migraine pathogenesis. In the future, medications that influence chaotic dynamics (such as glial cell modulators) may allow for a greater effect with less drug.*

By affecting chaotic (nonlinear) controls—whereby a tiny change in initial conditions may lead to a profound difference later in the process—new therapies may be employed that use less drug in the migraine cascade than is currently required.

The brain works primarily via synapses that interpret incoming inhibitory and excitatory impulses and nonlinear dynamics are involved in the feedback system of these complex neuronal systems. Physiologically, for energy conservation, it would make sense for living systems to utilize a nonlinear system, rather than random or simple linear dynamics. By utilizing a system where a tiny change in initial conditions may result in a major difference "downstream," a great deal of energy may be conserved. Chaos is a subset of nonlinear systems. Low-dimensional chaos theory may be the only way to explain how complex neurological systems are adaptable, efficient, versatile, and have effective feedback homeostasis. A large body of evidence has indicated that electrical activity of the brain, heart rhythms, blood glucose levels, and glycolysis are all governed, to some extent, by chaotic dynamics. Characteristics of chaotic systems include:

1. Extreme sensitivity to initial conditions; a tiny change upstream may lead to an enormous difference downstream. This would have major implications for headache therapies, as influencing the neuron's initial conditions would require much less drug than attempting to affect all of the components later in the cascade.
2. The deterministic, not random, nature of chaotic dynamics. Chaotic output of a deterministic system, when plotted, mimics randomness but is not random and, in that sense, "chaos" is a misnomer.
3. Chaotic systems possess a small number of independent variables, and the output is complex and deterministic.
4. The behavior of a system partially controlled by chaotic dynamics may change dramatically with a tiny change in the value of one parameter and is called a bifurcation.
5. The sequence of data in a chaotic system may be plotted and viewed as a phase space set.

To demonstrate chaotic mechanisms takes an enormous amount of data but this chapter will simply describe the possible role of chaotic dynamics in headache pathophysiology [27, 20].

## *Background*

Chaos is a math-based, nonlinear dynamical theory. Chaos has been used to predict the behavior of ion flow, as well as neural and biosystems. Chaos is a misnomer, as it is deterministic, not random. A key property is extreme sensitivity to initial conditions so that a tiny change in initial conditions results in huge changes downstream. This has advantages for biosystems, particularly in conserving energy. Chaos has been shown to govern the beating of the heart, as well as the evolution of epileptic seizures.

Ionic flow is governed by either random, linear, or chaotic (nonlinear) controls. Chaotic control means that a *small* change in the channel protein results in a *large* change in the channel protein shape. This saves energy as compared to a simple linear control system. Ionic dynamics are crucial in cortical spreading depression (CSD). A tiny change in $K^+$ efflux, or $Ca^+$ influx, will result in a large effect downstream, with CSD and oligemia. Chaos has been demonstrated to play a role in $K^+$, $Ca^+$, and $Na^+$ movements. Tiny perturbations—possibly brought about via weather, stress, or hormonal changes—in the hyperexcitable brain may result in CSD and eventually in PPE. Only chaotic dynamics could logically explain the cascade that leads from CSD to PPE.

The drugs that affect CSD may influence the membrane through chaotic controls. Drugs that better control chaos may inhibit CSD. For instance, by affecting $K^+$ efflux through small effects *upstream,* we may prevent the events *downstream* that lead to headache. This has been demonstrated to be true with epileptic seizures. Peripherally, the familiar cascade of $Mg^{++}$ binding to *N*-methyl-D-aspartate (NMDA), with subsequent $Ca^+$ influx, is very sensitive to initial conditions and changes. Drugs that work through chaotic controls peripherally may be effective in very small concentrations.

With central sensitization (CS), windup is a typical system that is probably controlled by a nonlinear flexible system (chaos). Linear dynamics could not explain or control windup. Different aspects of CS are most likely under chaotic control, from NMDA activation to nitric oxide synthesis. Thalamic recruitment involved in expansion of the pain area is best explained by chaos. The pathological shift of homeostasis seen in chronic CS, with a loss of brain stem inhibition, may actually reflect a *loss* of chaotic control. This is similar to the loss of control in the heart, resulting in v-tachycardia. The brain stem periaqueductal gray (PAG)—important in migraine—has been shown to be under chaotic control through P/Q-type $Ca^+$ channels. Chaos may assert its most profound effects in the brain stem.

## *Chaos and the Nervous System*

Chaotic dynamics has been proven to function at a variety of levels in the nervous system. Both individual neurons (particularly in squid giant axons), as well as in neuronal systems, have been shown to be—at least some of the time—governed by nonlinear dynamics. Neuronal networks of thalamocortical circuits have their feedback loops managed by chaotic dynamics. Neural network models in analyzing thalamic networks have demonstrated the presence of chaos. In a person with epilepsy, when chaos fails and patterns become too regular, an epileptic seizure may result to return brain dynamics to a more normal (chaotic) state. By the very nature of generators of complex neural behaviors, they cannot be random but must be deterministic and nonlinear, at least some of the time. It is likely that neuronal dynamics vacillate and totter between random, linear, and chaotic dynamics [27].

Chaos theory may help us understand why a patient experiences a severe headache associated with a weather change or other headache triggers

## *Chaos at the Ionic Level*

The flow of ions about the cell has been determined to be a combination of randomness, linear (deterministic) movements, and chaotic processes. Again, for energy saving, chaotic mechanisms are more efficient. Chaotic mechanisms in the brain stem may explain why tiny changes in weather or hormones may result in a migraine. Most neuronal activity in the brain stem involves postsynaptic inhibition that has been demonstrated to be governed by chaotic mechanisms. If we were dealing with a linear system, a tiny change in weather, stress, hormones, or sleep would not lead to neuronal activity differences. Chaotic dynamics will turn tiny initial changes or perturbations into major events, possibly triggering CSD. By altering the concentration of sodium outside of the cell, it has been demonstrated that the membrane response must be governed, at least in part, by chaos. Several studies have demonstrated chaos at the cellular level in the brain [44]. By utilizing the "jumps" of ions through the energy barriers of the channel protein, maps have been constructed that reveal the chaotic controls. Numerical solutions and algorithms have been constructed revealing when the transition to chaotic dynamics occurs [27].

Ion channel kinetics, partially controlled by chaotic dynamics, play a crucial role in CSD and in brain stem inhibition. A small change in the channel protein will result, through chaos, in a major difference in the shape of the protein. Neurons in the cortex fire with irregular patterns. Part of what governs the spiking patterns is the balance between excitatory and inhibitory inputs. The spiking patterns have been proven to be governed by chaotic dynamics, at least some of the time.

## *Chaos at the Neuronal Level*

Single neurons, as well as groups, fire in a variety of patterns, from regular oscillating patterns to bursts (and everything in between). Neurons, and neuronal systems, undergo transitions that carry them between diverse states [50]. Chaotic dynamics partially govern both individual neurons, as well as groups of neurons. The chaotic dynamics switch the neurons from one firing pattern to another. In the presence of low concentrations of serotonin, neuronal firing patterns change, with an increase in "beating" periods, all of which is consistent with chaotic dynamics. The synchronized dynamics of groups of neurons take the form, at times, of low-dimensional chaos. The presence of chaos has been proven to be a factor in the inhibitory synaptic noise of certain types of neurons. Experimental studies have shown that chaos is involved in the dynamics of central dopaminergic neuronal systems, particularly in the substantia nigra [40].

## CSD and Chaos

CSD induces calcium and sodium influx, with potassium efflux and P/Q calcium channels involved. It is much too delicate and complex to be run by a random mechanism or simple linear kinetics. Chaotic controls have been demonstrated to be involved with these channel ionic movements. Chaos would also aid in explaining some of the properties of CSD. The initiation of CSD may be brought about by a very tiny change in potassium—with activation of receptors and resulting in a large change downstream thus causing CSD and oligemia. With the potassium efflux under (partial) chaotic control, the chaos probably helps to regulate the increased cortical hyperactivity inherent in the brain of some migraineurs. There is evidence that the PAG may be partially controlled by chaotic dynamics.

A tiny cortical input may result in activation of the trigeminal nucleus caudalis, with resultant release of pro-inflammatory peptides and a release of glutamate. CSD leads to PPE, with a very small perturbation upstream leading to this cascade. Only chaotic dynamics may explain how this sequence may be possible. The drugs that affect CSD (topiramate, amitriptyline, sodium valproate) may influence chaotic dynamics through membrane effects. It requires significantly less drug to influence the system if chaos is involved versus a system that is primarily governed by linear (or random) dynamics. As is the situation with epileptic seizures, preventing the propagation of impulses upstream, through tiny ionic changes, may lead to less of the headache cascade downstream.

## Sensitization

The pathological shift of homeostasis that is observed with chronic CS and a loss of brain stem inhibitory activity may actually reflect a loss of chaotic control. This is similar to a loss of chaotic controls in the heart leading to certain arrhythmias, or with a loss of chaos leading to a seizure.

Glutamate is the most prevalent excitatory neurotransmitter in the brain and, along with calcium, is crucial in positive feedback processes. Glutamate has been shown to be directly involved in bidirectional communications between neurons and astrocytes. Research has demonstrated that glutamate feedback processes are critical in the generation of complex bursting oscillations in astrocytes. These glutamate-mediated events are likely to be involved in memory storage, epilepsy, and migraine. The control of this feedback process may well be, at least partially, enacted through chaotic control. Peripherally, the familiar cascade of magnesium binding to NMDA, with subsequent calcium influx, is very sensitive to minute initial changes [17]. Chaotic controls would help to explain the dynamics of peripheral sensitization. Drugs that may influence chaotic dynamics could work peripherally in very low concentrations.

Simple nonlinear dynamics could not possibly explain the phenomenon of wind-up. NMDA receptor activation, as well as thalamic recruitment, would best be explained if they were controlled by nonlinear membrane/ionic dynamics.

## *Controlling Chaotic Dynamics*

By utilizing and influencing chaotic dynamics, significantly less drug would have to be employed, versus the amount required to affect a linear system. Brain-derived neurotrophic factor (BDNF) is a neurotropin that modulates the excitability of neuronal membranes. One study utilized BDNF to affect hippocampal neurons. It has been demonstrated that the patterns of electrical activity in hippocampal neurons are governed, in part, by chaotic dynamics. The hippocampal electrical system is a deterministic, chaotic one, with a few degrees of freedom. This "neuronal chaos" may be sensitive to change by the application of small amounts of materials, such as BDNF, that influence temporal spiking. In this study, the application of BDNF to cultured hippocampal neurons enhanced the reliability of spike timing and resulted in more stereotyped firing patterns. It was felt that BDNF influenced chaos through effects on sodium at the membrane level. BDNF enhanced membrane conductance and thus stabilized the membrane. The application of BDNF affected the switching between periodic and aperiodic neuronal oscillations. BDNF has been linked to modulation of neuroplasticity. The BDNF application decreased irregularity of firing patterns by modulating neuronal outputs as well as inputs. The result was a BDNF-induced chaos stabilization. This experiment with BDNF was the first one to demonstrate a pharmacological stabilization of chaos at the neuronal level [12].

## *Practical Applications*

In several areas of medicine, practical applications for chaos-type mathematical models are beginning to emerge. One company, Vicor Technologies, Inc., is utilizing a device (the PD2i) to identify patients at high risk for sudden cardiac death. This unit employs chaos theory to determine risk. In addition, the company is developing a similar device, using chaotic dynamics, to evaluate the health of the autonomic nervous system in patients with diabetic neuropathy.

Chaos theory may help us understand why a patient experiences a severe headache associated with a weather change or other headache triggers. Tiny perturbations in a migraineur's delicate autonomic nervous system may lead, after the familiar cascade of migrainous physiological events, to a migraine.

A number of studies have been done to identify the role, if any, of patent foramen ovale (PFO) in migraine. There may be an association, albeit not yet clinically proven, between PFO and migraine. Two current headache trials in Europe and North America ("Premium" and "Prima") are blinded, sham-controlled PFO closure studies. If indeed an association is proven, chaos theory may help to explain the relationship between PFO and migraine. A tiny (downstream) change in blood flow may lead (upstream) to a migraine attack.

To apply chaotic dynamics to pain or headache, we will need a great deal of basic research. The potential exists to create drugs that may utilize chaotic dynamics. For instance, glial cells modulate much of what goes on in the CNS. Glial cells utilize a small amount of neurotransmitter to modulate a large number of neurons. Future medications that affect glial cells may be effective through chaotic dynamics.

## *Conclusion*

The physical dynamics involved at the neuronal level, both intra- and extra-cellular, are too complex to be explained via random, or even linear, dynamics. Chaotic dynamics certainly play a role, at least some of the time. It has been demonstrated that chaotic dynamics help to govern individual neurons as well as neural systems. One fundamental principal of chaotic dynamics, unlike simple linear systems, is that a tiny change in initial conditions may lead to a profound difference later in the process. Only chaotic dynamics may explain why a tiny change in weather, stress, hormones, or sleep may result in a migraine. Chaos has been demonstrated to be involved in heart rhythms. Chaotic dynamics may also explain why a PFO may result, upstream, in an increase in CSD and headache. It is possible that, by utilizing and affecting chaotic controls, new therapies may be employed that utilize less drug than is currently required. Note this is a version of an article that was originally published in *Practical Pain Management*, Vol. 10, May 2010.

## Suggested Reading


1. Aamodt AH, Stovner LJ, Langhammer A, Hagen K, Zwart JA (2007) Is headache related to asthma, hay fever, and chronic bronchitis? The Head-HUNT study. Headache 47(2):204–212
2. Bigal ME, Sheftell FD, Rapoport AM et al. (2002) Chronic daily headache in a tertiary care population: correlation between the international society criteria and propose revisions of criteria for chronic daily headache. Cephalagia 22:432–438
3. Blumenthal HJ (2001) Headaches and sinus disease. Headache 41(9):883–888
4. Bø SH, Davidsen EM, Gulbrandsen P et al (2009) Cerebrospinal fluid cytokine levels in migraine, tension-type headaches and cervicogenic headache. Cephalagia 29(3):365–372
5. Cuesta MC, Quintero L, Pons H, Suarez-Roca H (2002) Substance P and calcitonin gene-related peptide increase IL-1 beta, Il-6 and TNF-alpha secretion from human peripheral blood mononuclear cells. Neurochem Int 40(4):301–306
6. Damodaram S, Thalakoti S, Freeman SE et al (2009) Tonabersat inhibits trigeminal ganglion neuronal-satellite glial cell signaling. Headache 49(1):5–20

7. Diaz-Mitoma F, Vanast WJ, Tyrell DL (1987) Increased frequency of Epstein-Barr virus excretion in patients with new daily persistent headache. Lancet 1:411–415
8. Dimlich RV, Keller JT, Strauss TA, Fritts MJ (1991) Linear arrays of homogeneous mast cells in the dura matter of the rat. J Neurocytol 20(6):485–503
9. Eross E, Dodick D, Eross M (2007) The Sinus, Allergy, and Migraine Study (SAMS). Headache 47(2):213–224
10. Evans RW (2012) New daily persistent headache. Headache 52(S 1):40–44
11. Fu D, Guo Q, Ai Y et al. (2006) Glial activation and segmental upregulation of interleukin-*B* in the rat spinal cord after surgical incision. Neurochem Res 31:333–340
12. Fujisawa S, Yamada M, Nishiyama N, Ikegaya N (2004) BDNF boosts spike fidelity in chaotic neural oscillations. Biophys J 86(3):1820–1828
13. Gilman-Sachs A, Robbins L, Baum L (1989) Flow cytometric analysis of lymphocyte subsets in peripheral blood of chronic headache patients. Headache 29(5):290–294
14. Goadsby PJ (2011) New daily persistent headache: a symptom, not a discrete disorder. Headache 51:650–653
15. Hasselblatt M, Köhler J, Volles E, Ehrenreich H (1999) Simultaneous monitoring of endothelin-1 and vasopressin plasma levels in migraine. Neuroreport 10(2):423–425
16. Hotta K, Funahashi T, Arita Y et al (2000) Plasma concentrations of novel, adipose-specific protein, adiponectin, in type 2 diabetic patients. Atherioscler Thromb Vasc Biol 20(6):1595–1599
17. Kernick D (2005) Migraine—new perspectives from chaos theory. Cephalalgia 25:561–566
18. King R, Barchas J, Huberman B (1984) Chaotic behavior in dopamine neurodynamics. Proc Natl Acad Sci USA 81(4):1244–1247
19. Koenig MA, Gladstein J, McCarter RJ et al (2002) Chronic daily headache in children and adolescents presenting to tertiary headache clinics. Headache 42:491–500
20. Korn H, Faure P (2003) Is there chaos in the brain? C R Biologies 326:787–840
21. Koulchitsky S, Fischer MJM, Messlinger K (2009) Calcitonin gene-related peptide receptor inhibition reduces neuronal activity induced by prolonged increase in nitric oxide in the rat spinal trigeminal nucleus. Cephalagia 29(4):408–417
22. Lassen LH, Haderslev PA, Jacobsen VB, Iversen HK, Sperling B, Olesen J (2002) CGRP may play a causative role in migraine. Cephalagia 22(1):54–61
23. Levite M (1998) Neuropeptides, by direct interaction with T-cells, induce cytokine secretion and break the commitment to a distant T helper phenotype. Proc Natl Acad Sci U S A 95:12544–12549
24. Levy D, Burstein R, Kainz V, Jakubowski M, Strassman AM (2007) Mast cell degranulation activates a pain pathway underlying migraine headache. Pain 1330(1–2):166–176
25. Liberski PP, Mirecka B (1984) Mast cells in cluster headache: ultra-structure, release pattern and possible pathogenetic significance. Cephalagia 4(2):101–106
26. Li J, Vause CV, Durham PL (2008) Calcitonin gene-related peptide stimulation of nitric oxide synthesis and release from trigeminal ganglion glial cells. Brain Res 1196:22–32
27. Liebovitch L (1998) Fractals and chaos: simplified for the life sciences. Oxford University Press, New York
28. Lipton RB, Diamond S, Reed M, Diamond ML, Stewart WF (2001) Migraine diagnosis and treatment: results of the American Migraine Study II. Headache 41(7):638–645
29. Low NC, Merikangas KR (2003) The comorbidity of migraine. CNS Spectr 8(6):433–444
30. Mortimer MJ, Kay J, Gawkrodger DJ, Jaron A, Barker DC (1993) The prevalence of headache and migraine in atopic children: An epidemiological study in general practice. Headache 33(8):427–431
31. Moskovitz P, Cooper M (2010) Activated Glia: targets for the treatment of neuropathic pain. Pract Pain Manag 10(9):78–84
32. Ozge A, Ozge C, Ozturk C et al (2006) The relationship between migraine and atopic disorders-the contribution of pulmonary function tests and immunological screening. Cephalalgia 26(2):172–179

33. Peng KP, Fuh JL, Yuan HK et al (2001) New daily persistent headache: should migrainous features be incorporated? Cephalagia 31:1561–1569
34. Perini F, D'Andrea G, Galloni E, Pignatelli F, Billo G, Alba S, Bussone G, Toso V (2005) Plasma cytokine levels in migraineurs and controls. Headache 45(7):926–931
35. Peterlin BL, Bigl ME, Tepper SJ, Urakaze M, Sheftell FD, Rapoport AM (2007) Migraine and adiponectin: is there a connection? Cephalagia 27:435–446
36. Prakash S, Shah, ND (2010) Postinfectious new daily persistent headache may respond to intravenous methylprednisone. J Headache Pain 11(1):59–66
37. Robbins MS, Grosberg BM, Napchan U et al (2002) Clinical and prognostic subforms of new daily persistent headache. Cephalagia 22:66–69
38. Robbins L, Maides J, Shmaryan D (2009) The immune system and headache: a review. Pain Pract 19(3):47–51
39. Rozen TD (2011) New daily persistent headache: clinical perspective. Headache 51:641–649
40. Rozen TD, Swidan S (2006) Elevation of CSF tumor necrosis factor alpha levels in NDPH and treatment of refractory chronic daily migraine. Headache 46:897
41. Rozen T, Swidan SZ (2007) Elevation of CSF tumor necrosis factor alpha levels in new daily persistent headache and treatment-refractory chronic migraine. Headache 47(7):1050–1055
42. Rozen TD, Roth JM, Denenberg N (2005) Joint hypermobility as a predisposing factor for the development of new daily persistent headache. Headache 45:828–829
43. Sarchielli P, Alberti A, Baldi A et al (2006) Proinflammatory cytokines, adhesion molecules, and lymphocyte integrin expression in the internal jugular blood of migraine patients without aura assessed ictally. Headache 46(2):200–207
44. Schweighofer N, Doya K et al (2004) Chaos may enhance transmission in the inferior olive. Proc Natl Acad Sci USA 101(13):4655–4660
45. Tepper SJ, Stillman MJ (2008) Clinical and pre-clinical rationale for CGRP-receptor antagonists in the treatment of migraine. Headache 48(8):1259–1268
46. Thalakoti S, Patil VV, Damodaram S, Vause CV, Langford LE, Freeman SE et al (2007) Neuron-glia signaling in trigeminal ganglion; implications for migraine pathology. Headache 47(7):1008–1023
47. Thonnard-Neumann E (1977) Migraine therapy with heparin: pathophysiologic basis. Headache 16(6):284–292
48. Thonnard-Neumann E, Neckers LM (1981) T-Lymphocytes in migraine. Ann Allergy 47(4):325–332
49. Vale ML, Marques JB, Moreira CA et al (2003) Antinociceptive effects of interleukin-4, -10, and -13 on the writhing response in mice and zymosan-induced knee joint incapacitation in rats. J Pharmacol Exp Ther 304:102–108
50. Vreeswijk C, Sompolinsky H (1998) Chaos in neuronal networks with balanced excitatory and inhibitory activity. Science 274:1724–1726
51. Wagner R, Myers RR (1996) Endoneurial injection of TNF-alpha produces neuropathic pain behaviors. Neuroreport 7:2897–2901
52. Wilkinson IA, Halliday JA, Henry RL, Hankin RG, Hensley MJ (1994) Headache and asthma. J Pediatr Child Health 30:253–256
53. Wintrich S, Rothner D (2012) New daily persistent headaches—follow up and outcome in children and adolescents. Headache 50:s23
54. Yao MZ, Gu JF, Wang JH et al (2002) Interleukin-2 gene therapy of chronic neuropathic pain. Neuroscience 112(2):409–416

# Index




L. Robbins, *Advanced Headache Therapy,* DOI 10.1007/978-3-319-13899-2

CPSIA information can be obtained at www.ICGtesting.com
Printed in the USA
LVOW01s2151130515

438454LV00005B/28/P